UNPAID WORK IN NURSING HOMES

UNPAID WORK IN NURSING HOMES

Flexible Boundaries

Edited by
Pat Armstrong

First published in Great Britain in 2023 by

Policy Press, an imprint of
Bristol University Press
University of Bristol
1–9 Old Park Hill
Bristol
BS2 8BB
UK
t: +44 (0)117 374 6645
e: bup-info@bristol.ac.uk

Details of international sales and distribution partners are available at
policy.bristoluniversitypress.co.uk

British Library Cataloguing in Publication Data

A catalogue record for this book is available from the British Library

ISBN 978-1-4473-6616-4 paperback
ISBN 978-1-4473-6617-1 ePub
ISBN 978-1-4473-6618-8 ePdf

Cover design: Robin Hawes
Front cover image: iStock/shuoshu
Bristol University Press and Policy Press use environmentally responsible print partners.
Printed and bound in Great Britain by CPI Group (UK) Ltd, Croydon, CR0 4YY

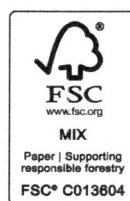

Contents

Notes on contributors

Gudmund Ågotnes is Associate Professor in the Department of Welfare and Participation at Western Norway University of Applied Sciences in Bergen, Norway. His research interests include mechanisms for inclusion, marginalisation and cohesion, participatory democratic processes and methods, and the relationship between government service design and civil society. Selected publications: 'Perspectives on migrant care workers in the long-term care sector: Identity politics and othering' (2022), *Nordic Journal of Migration Research*; 'From volunteer work to informal care by stealth: A "new voluntarism" in social democratic health and welfare services for older adults?' (2022), *Ageing & Society*.

Hugh Armstrong is Distinguished Research Professor Emeritus at the School of Social Work at Carleton University in Ottawa, Canada. Dr Armstrong's research interests include political economy of health, long-term care, and women and work. Selected publications: *The Privatization of Care: The Case of Nursing Homes*, edited with Pat Armstrong (2020), Routledge; 'Policies and practices: The case of RAI-MDS in Canadian long-term care homes' (2016), *Journal of Canadian Studies*.

Pat Armstrong is Distinguished Research Professor Emerita in the Department of Sociology at York University in Toronto, Canada, and a Fellow of the Royal Society of Canada. Dr Armstrong's research focuses on social policy, women and work, women's health, health care and long-term care. Selected publications: 'Is there a future for nursing homes in Canada?' (2021), *Healthcare Management Forum*; *Creative Teamwork*, edited with Ruth Lowndes (2018), Oxford University Press; *Wash, Wear and Care: Clothing and Laundry in Long-Term Residential Care*, with Suzanne Day (2017), McGill-Queen's University Press.

Susan Braedley is Associate Professor at the School of Social Work at Carleton University in Ottawa, Canada. Dr Braedley's feminist-political-economy-informed research programme explores the relationship between care work and capitalism in the context of socio-demographic aging, global migration and welfare state austerity policies. Selected publication: 'We're told, "Suck it up": Long-term care workers' psychological health and safety' (2017), *Ageing International*.

Jacqueline Choiniere is Associate Professor at the School of Nursing in the Faculty of Health at York University in Toronto, Canada. Dr Choiniere's research focuses on the influence of political, economic and social forces on the quality of care and on the quality of work and life for nurses and other health-care providers, including in settings where older adults receive care. Selected publication: 'Mapping nursing home inspections & audits in six countries', with Malcolm Doupe et al (2016), *Ageing International.*

Frode F. Jacobsen is Professor and Research Director at the Centre for Care Research at Western Norway University of Applied Sciences in Bergen, Norway. Dr Jacobsen's recent research has primarily been in the field of older people's care, both in a national and an international comparative perspective. Selected publication: 'Informal use of restraint in nursing homes: A threat to human rights or necessary care to preserve residents' dignity?' (2020), *Health.*

Janna Klostermann is Assistant Professor in the Department of Sociology of the University of Calgary in Calgary, Canada. Dr Klostermann is a feminist sociologist and long-term care scholar exploring the politics of care through narrative, ethnographic and arts-based research. 'What about the limits of care?' is a question central to her work. She is a member of the research team working on the project 'Changing Places: Unpaid Work in Public Places' . Her work has recently appeared in *Ageing & Society* and *Societies.*

Ruth Lowndes is Research Associate at the Department of Sociology at York University in Toronto, Canada. Dr Lowndes is currently doing research into long-term care within the 'COVID-19, Families and Long-term Residential Care' and 'Changing Places: Unpaid Work in Public Spaces' projects led by Dr Pat Armstrong. She is also registered with the College of Nurses of Ontario and is a certified diabetes educator. Selected publication: 'Social participation in long-term residential care: Case studies from Canada, Norway and Germany' with James Struthers and Gudmund Ågotnes (2020), *Canadian Journal on Aging.*

Oddrunn Sortland received her doctorate from the University of Bergen in cooperation with the Center for Care Research at Western Norway University of Applied Sciences in Bergen, Norway. Her expertise is in the areas of family care, primary care nursing, community nursing, nursing education and geriatric nursing. Selected publication: 'Shared care and organizing help to older people living at home: A field of tensions between the elderly, the family and home care services' in S. Glasdam and F. Jacobsen (eds) (2020) *When the Aged Human Gets Ill or Impaired,* Gads Forlag.

Christine Streeter is a PhD candidate at the School of Social Work at Carleton University in Ottawa, Canada. She is involved in research that explores gender, work and labour, and is committed to improving insecure working conditions for care workers in the social work and social services work sectors. Her most recent work includes a report on safety for LGBTQ2+ older adults and workers in public services, published in 2020 by the Canadian Union of Public Employees and Egale. Her dissertation analyses conditions of work and care in the non-profit and social service sectors both before the COVID-19 pandemic and during it.

James Struthers is Professor Emeritus of Canadian Studies at Trent University in Peterborough in Ontario, Canada. Dr Struthers' research interests include the history of Canadian social policy in the areas of unemployment, social assistance, old age pensions, home care and long-term residential care. Selected publications include: 'Home, hotel, hospital, hospice: Conflicting images of long-term residential care in Ontario, Canada', in Sally Chivers and Ulla Kriebernegg (eds) *Care Home Stories: Aging, Disability, and Long-Term Residential Care* (2017) transcript Verlag; and *The Limits of Affluence: Welfare in Ontario, 1920–1970* (1994), University of Toronto Press.

Marta Szebehely is Professor Emeritus at the Department of Social Work at Stockholm University in Sweden. Dr Szebehely is involved in international comparative research on eldercare, and analyses how policy and organisational changes in eldercare have affected the everyday life of care workers, and of older people with care needs and their family members. Research interests include theories of care, care policies, gender and work organisation.

Petra Ulmanen is Assistant Professor at the Department of Social Work at Stockholm University in Sweden. Her main research areas are social care, and social policy and gender, primarily focusing on family caregiving for older persons and its social and economic consequences. Selected publications: 'Reversed socioeconomic pattern in the costs of caring regarding well-being and paid work among women in Sweden' (2021), *Social Policy and Administration*; 'From the state to the family or to the market? Consequences of reduced residential eldercare in Sweden' with Marta Szebehely (2015), *International Journal of Social Welfare*.

Acknowledgements

We would like to acknowledge at least five essential ingredients making this book possible:

First, our extraordinary, committed, interdisciplinary, international research team has dedicated hundreds and hundreds of hours for more than a decade to making nursing homes as good as they can be. While only some of us have names on the chapters in this book, every chapter reflects our collective work.

Second, this book is only possible because those who live in, work in, visit, and manage nursing homes trusted us to share their stories and analysis with us and because our partners from unions and the employer community provided us with information along with continual feedback on and analysis of our research. We hope this book affirms their trust.

Third, funding from the Social Science and Humanities Research Council of Canada as well as from the Canadian Institutes of Health Research and the European Research Area in Ageing 2, has made it possible for us both to continue to build on and expand our knowledge and to share it with and beyond academe.

Fourth, we are kept organised, on time and on budget by the totally indispensable Wendy Winters and our books are ensured readability with Jane Springer's excellent editing.

Fifth, Policy Press has provided continual support in getting this book to the public.

Introduction: framing and comparing unpaid care work

Pat Armstrong and Marta Szebehely

'Nursing home', 'care home' and 'long-term care home' are all terms used for places that are intended to provide 24-hour paid care, primarily for older people. In high-income countries, these residential places provide the largest portion of long-term care for those defined as unable to care for themselves and for whom hospital care is not required. The demand for a place in these homes is increasing rapidly, as more people live into old age with complex care needs that cannot be handled at home, even with paid support and assistance from unpaid family and friends.

Nursing homes vary considerably in size, funding, staffing and organisation, but they all provide support for the activities of daily living, as well as nursing care. And in all of them, the paid care is provided primarily by women for women, with many of the women doing the work racialised and/or newcomers. However, when someone moves into a nursing home, the unpaid care work previously provided by family, friends and volunteers does not necessarily disappear. New forms of unpaid labour may be required and the type of unpaid labour required may change over time with public policies, individual residents' health, and other developments, such as COVID-19. It is not only family and friends who do this unpaid work in nursing homes, though. Residents continue to do some forms of unpaid work for themselves and may take on new labour for other residents. Volunteers, too, do some of the care work in these homes. In addition, those formally employed in the home take on additional work without pay to fill the gaps in what they see as necessary care.

The pandemic put a spotlight on long-term care and especially on nursing homes, where so many died from COVID-19, drawing particular attention to the many non-employees who enter nursing homes daily. Banning visitors was a key response to COVID throughout the high-income countries until it became obvious that banning visitors for residents was 'detrimental to their well-being' (Curry and Langins, 2020). Strategies were rapidly developed to maintain contact with 'essential caregivers', a term for people who are not paid for their necessary care work.

Although the work of social support and social connecting long provided by families and friends became particularly visible and valued during the pandemic, less attention was paid to the full range of unpaid work they and others do. Largely invisible too were the variations across and within jurisdictions in what work is defined as essential; in who does the work, and under what conditions; in who feels responsible, and who is held responsible; and with what the consequences are.

In this book, we focus on uncovering the extent and nature of unpaid work and workers in nursing homes. Understanding these activities as work allows us to explore the conditions and relations that shape them, while attending to the multiple skills and tensions involved as well as to the values and structures that shape them.

The guiding theory

Feminist political economy, which guides the research in this book, seeks to make visible the multiple forces, relations and conditions that shape lives. It asks who benefits and who does not, in what ways, when, and with what consequences for individuals and collectives. It begins by investigating how a society provides for food, shelter, jobs and joy, and for daily as well as generational reproduction through both paid and unpaid work (Luxton, 1980; Armstrong and Armstrong, 1990). From this perspective, the search for profit shapes but does not determine this provision, and people make their own history, although not under conditions of their own choosing. Values also matter, with values understood as both a consequence of how things are done and a cause of how they are done.

Feminists are particularly interested in care work, work primarily done by women in all societies. This means thinking through why gender in all its intersections matters, how it matters and for whom, with the intent of developing strategies building towards social justice. This includes understanding care as a relationship (Bourgault and Robinson, 2019), albeit frequently an unequal one in terms of power, knowledge, capacities and the right to care.

For us, care in these homes encompasses not only emotional support, social support and connections, along with coordination, management, diagnosis, medical treatment and personal care. It also includes a clean environment and clean clothes, nutritional food, stimulating activities and appropriate supplies. It extends to advocacy, education, communication and worries about both the residents and the care provided.

All this requires skilled work based on experience as well as training, much of which is informal and the result of women learning and working together (Armstrong, 2013; Barken and Armstrong, 2017). Nevertheless, care work has often been portrayed as something women do 'naturally', by virtue of being female, and thus something that requires little skill (Baines et al, 2017), especially when it comes to activities long associated with daily living, like bathing. Such an assumption helps to justify having care work provided by those unpaid and untrained for the job.

Feminist political economy is always a theory in process, and research is a dialogue between theory and evidence (Thompson, 1978), with theory guiding where and how to look but always shaped by the emerging evidence. Theory is assessed and altered by listening to the voices of those who do the work, as Dorothy Smith (1987) encouraged us to do. Our feminist approach means continually sharing and debating data collection and analysis within our international, interdisciplinary, intergenerational research team.

Some of our most vulnerable people live and work in nursing homes, or visit them. They are a barometer of the economic, political, cultural and social conditions, as well as of values. They thus raise issues that go well beyond specific services and practices: issues such as fundamental human and social rights; systemic discrimination; the role of the state and of profit; the responsibilities of individuals, families, markets and governments; work organisation and skills; and approaches to care.

For us, context matters, and it matters at multiple levels. While nursing homes across high-income countries share some common characteristics, they also display significant diversity. We seek to understand complexity in care organisation and in care relationships, which are often characterised by inequities, leading us to include all those who live in, work in, visit and manage nursing homes. This means capturing tensions and contradictions – such as those between medical and social care, families and staff providing care, safety and risk, choice and compulsion, and paid and unpaid work – and seeing them as ongoing and thus requiring recognition and handling.

From this perspective, these places for care are both homes and workplaces. How work is funded, organised, managed and staffed has a direct impact on the boundaries between paid and unpaid work. We assume that the conditions of work are the conditions of care, whether the work is done for pay or not. And a labour of love is still labour. Many feel rewarded by such work, but it is often a form of 'compulsory altruism', especially for women, as Hilary Land and Hilary Rose (1985) made clear long ago.

Our approach guides us to locate specific experiences of individuals and groups in nursing homes within the context of the local, national and international political economies, always recognising that gender in all its intersections matter. In doing so, we seek to capture the complexities and contradictions that are critical to understanding how things work.

The evidence

The empirical basis for the chapters in this book comes from a long series of comparative studies on nursing homes. Our team began doing comparative research on nursing homes nearly 20 years ago with a survey of staff in four Nordic countries and four Canadian provinces. Our research revealed significant differences in the experiences of the staff, even though the resident populations were quite similar across the countries. For example, the Canadian participants were more than six times as likely as their Nordic counterparts to say they experienced violence on a more or less daily basis (Armstrong et al, 2009). That research prompted our ten-year project titled 'Reimagining Long-term Residential Care: An International Study in Promising Practices'. Completed in 2020, the project brought together academics and students from a wide range of disciplines, along with our partners from unions, employer organisations and a community group, to study nursing homes in Canada, Germany, Norway, Sweden, the UK and the US, capturing approaches from jurisdictions that reflected the three forms of welfare states described by Esping-Andersen (1990) – liberal, conservative and social democratic. What we learned about unpaid work, not only from that large project but also from multiple others the project spawned for our team members, led to our current project, 'Changing Places: Unpaid Work in Public Places'. While we draw on our research in six countries for this book, as well as on our other projects, our focus here is on Canada, Norway and Sweden. That early survey, along with our continuing work, revealed for us the significant contrasts between Nordic and Canadian approaches to nursing homes that allow us to draw lessons for theory, policy and practices. At the same time, we can also learn from differences between two social democratic countries as well as from urban–rural differences within them. We provide more details on these different contexts in the next section.

Our mixed methods are described in *Creative Teamwork: Developing Rapid, Site-switching Ethnography* (Armstrong and Lowndes [eds] 2018). In brief, we undertook analytical mapping on the basis of literature reviews and both statistical and policy data analysis to provide a complex picture of nursing homes in each of the jurisdictions. We also identified larger structural issues at the global, national and local levels, related to issues such as funding and ownership. The many products of this work can be found at https://reltc. apps01.yorku.ca/. Updating that analysis for this book with new research on policy and structural changes prompted by the pandemic, we set the context that shapes unpaid work in each jurisdiction.

New ethnographic methods we have developed provided a major source of data and analysis for the larger study, for our other projects, and for the current one, which focuses on urban and rural homes in the three countries. For our big project, we took international, interdisciplinary, intergenerational teams of researchers into care homes over the course of a week so that we could interview, observe and reflect together on what we saw and heard. Teams worked in pairs and in shifts, beginning before 7 am and ending after midnight. The approach brought 'fresh eyes' to the research, with all teams including both those familiar with the jurisdiction and those new to it. We used similar techniques, on a smaller scale, for 'Changing Places', as well as for our other projects that inform this work. Our larger study included 24 homes, 'Changing Places' added six more, and an additional ten sites have been studied in our other shared projects. The homes we studied varied in size and ownership, but all received considerable public funding and in all homes the majority of residents and workers were women. They thus reflected the range of homes found in all the countries we studied. Drawing primarily on the sites in Canada, Norway and Sweden, we highlight the implications for theory, policy and practices, illustrating what we have learned from these decades of research through direct references to these studies, at the same time as our qualitative work provides the basic data for our analysis.

Each of the chapters in this book is written by a specific author or set of authors, but the data and analysis are the result of our collective work. Indeed, all of our work reflects our practice of gathering, sharing and reflecting together on our research and analysis.

The context for unpaid care

The number of people living into old age has been growing for years. Although the majority are healthy and live independently, more people are surviving into old age with multiple complex care needs. The aging population in all three countries has increased the demand for care, care that requires considerable skill. Governments in these countries have responded with different kinds and amounts of public care. Neoliberal approaches that promote greater reliance on markets, on free trade, on for-profit strategies and services, and on individual responsibility for care have had an impact on care in all the countries we studied. There are, however, differences among the countries in the extent to which they have embraced neoliberalism.

In all three countries, paid and unpaid care is primarily the responsibility of women. At the same time, there are differences in who does what kind of work and how they are formally prepared for that work, with important implications for unpaid care.

Normative frameworks

Unpaid care work is shaped by values about the right to care and who is responsible for providing care, as well as by access to nursing homes and to alternatives, such as home care. All three countries support universal access to and collective responsibility for health care, with some important differences. When it comes to care for the older population in our three countries, Norway displays the greatest commitment to the principle of universality and Canada the least.

The Scandinavian countries have been labelled universalistic 'caring states' or 'social services states' because of their generously funded, publicly provided care services offered to and used by all social groups (Leira, 1994; Anttonen, 2002). Building Scandinavian universality after World War II was based on the understanding that services should not only be publicly funded but publicly provided. Only a democratically steered public sector was seen as capable of guaranteeing equal access to the same high-quality services for both rich and poor.

However, compared to other, more equitable welfare services, long-term care for older people in Norway and Sweden has been characterised by a weak form of universalism: the legal right to services is limited and services can be accessed only after needs assessment by local gatekeepers, who are circumscribed by tight municipal budgets. Although the commitment to equity remains in legislation and policy documents, without changes in policies or legislation to respond to emerging demands, in practice long-term care is not universal. A weak form of universalism has become increasingly weaker in both Norway and Sweden (Kröger, 2003; Szebehely and Meagher, 2018).

Home-care services and care homes are increasingly targeted at those with the most complex care needs. Almost one third of Swedish care home places have disappeared since the year 2000. Today 4 per cent of the population aged 65 years and older live in a care home; this is a decline from 8 per cent. Despite declining coverage, Norway has more care home beds: 6 per cent of the population aged 65 years and older live in a care home (Swedish Agency for Health and Care Services, 2021, pp 102–3).

Home care has a long history in Scandinavia (Szebehely and Meagher, 2018). Applications for residential care may be turned down with the argument that the needs can be met by intensive home care instead. Most people who move to a Swedish care home have received a considerable amount of home care before the move (National Board of Health and Welfare, 2019). Differing definitions of care make it difficult to compare the use of home care, but available data indicate that a higher proportion receive home care in Norway, although the intensity of care is higher in Sweden (Szebehely and Meagher, 2018).

Particularly in Sweden, home care has become increasingly predefined, time-squeezed and fragmented. Continuity is low, with a large number of workers involved in each client's care (Strandell, 2020). As a result, home care has become less attractive over time and care homes have become more desirable.

The Canadian system for hospital and doctor care is also based on universalism, shared responsibility, and the right to care but it is primarily public payment for care, rather than public provision (Naylor, 1986). With the expansion of feeless services from the 1960s, many older people gained access to hospital care, which meant there was limited demand for extensive care in nursing homes.

In Canada, health care is primarily a provincial and territorial responsibility and neither home care nor long-term care fall under the federal legislation requiring universality. All the jurisdictions provide public funds for nursing homes and all charge regulated fees that are kept low enough to ensure access. However, there is considerable variation across jurisdictions (Armstrong and Armstrong, 2016). Given this diversity, we focus here on Ontario, Canada's most populated province, to provide a specific example of unpaid care in nursing homes.

As James Struthers (2017) explains, in the 1960s a combination of overflowing hospitals, women's growing labour force participation, housing shortages, and the exposure of terrible conditions in private nursing homes led to the rapid expansion of public and charitably owned care homes. They were promoted as 'the best place in the community for his care and comfort', places that were intended to provide 'a public service available to everyone' (Struthers, 2017, pp 288–9).

All this changed with neoliberal policies, beginning in the 1970s. The federal government cut back its contribution to hospital care, prompting Ontario to significantly reduce the number of acute care hospital beds, and close chronic care and many mental health hospitals. This left older people seeking care elsewhere. Nursing home places did not keep up with demand, producing long waiting lists for entry for those deemed eligible under rigid criteria. OECD data indicate that about 4 per cent of [Canadians] aged 65 and over are in long-term care (OECD, 2021, p 261). If retirement homes and assisted living are excluded, the number is closer to 3 per cent. Families and individuals are held primarily responsible for older people's care in both policy and practice.

There has been some publicly funded home care offered in Ontario since the 1970s. There are no public data on how many hours individuals actually receive but it is clear that the hours are much lower in practice than the allowed 14 hours a week. Families still provide 80 per cent of home care, with a quarter of them providing 40 hours of unpaid care a week (Home Care Ontario, nd). Home care in Ontario is 'understaffed, underfunded and inequitable in access to care ' (Yakerson, 2019, p 260), with limited continuity in services, especially in those provided by the publicly funded for-profit companies which deliver most of the care.

In sum, there are significant differences in attitudes towards nursing homes among the three jurisdictions. Despite inadequate home care, opinion polls indicate that more than 90 per cent of Ontarians would prefer care at home (Home Care Ontario, nd). In contrast, a Swedish survey found the majority would prefer residential care if they needed help with personal care, rather than receiving home care several times a day (Szebehely, 2017). These differences reflect and are reflected in funding, ownership, staffing and the structures of nursing homes.

Funding and ownership

Funding indicates and influences values at the same time as it shapes unpaid care. This is also the case with marketisation, especially when it comes to ownership and the adoption of for-profit managerial strategies.

All Scandinavian countries have been affected by marketisation, albeit to different degrees. Before 1990, there was no for-profit nursing home ownership. While nine in ten nursing home beds in Norway and eight in ten in Sweden are still publicly owned, 18 per cent in Sweden and 2 per cent in Norway are operated by for-profit companies, mainly large corporations. Non-profit private providers have a limited role in both countries (operating 7 per cent of beds in Norway and 3 per cent in Sweden). In this respect long-term care is more universal in Norway than in Sweden (Ågotnes et al, 2019; National Board of Health and Welfare, 2022; Statistics Norway, 2022, Table 1).

In terms of funding, Scandinavian long-term care is still more universal than in many countries. In 2019, long-term care expenditure accounted for 3.7 per cent of GDP in Norway and 3.6 per cent in Sweden, compared to 2 per cent in Canada and 1.5 per cent on average across the OECD countries (OECD, 2021, p 269). However, in both Norway and Sweden, the share of GDP spent on long-term care for older people has declined, despite a rapidly aging population (Szebehely and Meagher, 2018).

Beginning in the 1990s, funding policies in Ontario made for-profit homes eligible for the same per diem public payment as other homes, and a competitive system for allocating new publicly funded places favours large, for-profit homes (Armstrong et al, 2016). Almost 60 per cent of Ontario nursing homes are owned by the for-profit sector and a majority of residents live in for-profit care homes. Only 16 per cent are government-owned, with the rest owned by non-profit private organisations (CIHI, 2021).

In sum, the Scandinavian countries spend more than Canada on nursing homes, and Ontario has gone the farthest in marketising care. According to the Ontario Long-term Care Commission (Marrocco et al, 2021, pp 38–9), for-profit nursing homes are of lower quality and provide less care, which helps explain why more Ontarians resist nursing homes and more Scandinavians prefer them.

Staffing

The most obvious impact of funding is on staffing and working conditions. The difference in spending between Canada and Scandinavia is reflected in the latter's higher number of long-term care workers per resident. However, neoliberal managerial approaches that promote more precarious work and working conditions are having an impact in all three countries.

Estimates indicate that staffing levels in Scandinavian care homes are two to three times higher than in Canada (Harrington et al, 2012). On average, in a Swedish care home, there are 3.3 residents per care worker on weekdays during the day, and 4 residents per worker on weekends (Szebehely, 2020).

Ontario residents average 2 hours and 45 minutes of care per day each (Marrocco et al, 2021, p 49), well below the minimum of the 4.1 hours recommended more than a decade ago, when care needs were less complex (Harrington et al, 2020). For-profit homes have lower staffing levels, bringing down the average. Publicly owned homes spend 81 per cent of their funds on wages and benefits but for-profits spend only 71 per cent (Ontario, 2020, p 10).

These figures represent scheduled staffing, not the actual number of people at work each day. Our 2005 survey data indicate that 46 per cent of care home workers in Norway and 42 per cent in Sweden worked in under-staffed premises at least once a week because their colleagues were off sick or absent for some other reason – a problem even more common in Canada, where 46 per cent experienced working in under-staffed situations more or less daily (Armstrong, et al, 2009, p 59).

There are some clear jurisdictional differences in the mix of staff skills. The way data are compiled and differences in required education make precise comparisons difficult. Registered nurses (RNs) are the most comparable. In Norway RNs account for 32 per cent of the workforce, compared to 8 per cent in Ontario and 6 per cent in Sweden. Staff with at least one year of formal training include the 44 per cent of health care workers in Norway, the 59 per cent of assistant nurses in Sweden and the 17 per cent of registered practical nurses in Ontario. Ontario relies most heavily on those with limited formal training, with personal support workers, who have a minimum of six months' training, accounting for nearly 60 per cent of the workforce (Ontario, 2020, p 14). Similar groups of care workers with short or no formal training (care aides) correspond to 33 and 21 per cent, respectively, of the Swedish and Norwegian care workforce (Swedish Agency for Health and Care Services, 2021).

Not only does skill mix differ among the countries, so too does the division of labour. In Sweden, most care workers do similar tasks – personal care, cleaning, laundry, social activities, documentation, contact with health-care professionals and the families of residents, handing out medication, and other medical tasks on delegation by RNs. With more RNs, Norway has a more detailed division of labour, based on training. The division of labour is most hierarchical in Ontario homes, where personal support workers have a much more limited range of tasks than a Swedish care aide and normally do not undertake medical tasks or take responsibility for contacting health-care professionals (Daly and Szebehely, 2012). Moreover, in Ontario, dietary aides, laundry workers and housekeepers, many of whom work for contracted companies, do tasks performed by Swedish care aides or assistant nurses. As a result, these contracted workers are not part of the care team and care is more fragmented for residents. In most Swedish and Norwegian homes, each resident has a contact person responsible for setting up the resident's care plan and for keeping in touch with the resident's family. Such a designated contact person is much less common in Ontario.

Although the skill mix and division of labour differ, employment conditions modelled on neoliberal principles are becoming increasingly similar and problematic in all three countries. A high proportion of care workers work part time: 62 per cent in Norway and 52 per cent in Sweden (OECD, 2021, p 265). In Ontario, 48 per cent of the personal support workers work part time, and 11 per cent are casuals (Ontario, 2020, p 5). Casual work is even more common in Sweden, where 28 per cent of the care home workers are employed by the hour (Szebehely, 2020, p 74). Arduous working conditions may force workers to 'choose' part-time work involuntarily, but in all three countries research shows that part-time staff want to work more hours (Drange and Vabø, 2021).

A 2005 survey of residential care workers indicated clearly that Scandinavians were better off than their Canadian counterparts regarding workload and both physical and psychological exhaustion at the end of the workday (Armstrong et al, 2009; Daly and Szebehely, 2012). However, a 2015 replication of the survey in the Nordic countries shows that conditions for Swedish care workers have deteriorated. The workload is heavier, and physical and psychological exhaustion have increased. In 2005 in Sweden, 40 per cent of residential care workers had seriously considered quitting – a proportion that increased to 50 per cent in 2015. Residential care workers have the highest level of sick leave of all occupational groups in Sweden (Stranz and Szebehely, 2018). In Ontario, a 2020 study showed that half of personal support workers leave within five years and 43 per cent left as a result of burnout caused by working in short-staffed situations (Ontario, 2020, p 6).

Norwegian care workers have seen less deterioration in their working conditions, and are less dissatisfied with their wages and less prone to leave their job. The more limited for-profit provision of care in Norway is likely an important factor, because considering quitting is more common in the private sector (Van Aerschot et al, 2022). However, in both Norway and Sweden, care workers are worried about their health and well-being at work and they feel undervalued by municipal leaders, which is clearly correlated with considering quitting (Elstad and Vabø, 2021). Although

Norwegian workers have better working conditions than workers in many other countries, care work in Norway is still a demanding occupation and not highly valued.

In Ontario, a focus on a limited number of tasks comes with for-profit ownership. The tasks considered most essential are medical ones, and the focus on them often leaves little room for social support. Concerns about quality raised in inspection, in the media and by families lead to more regulation of staff and more reporting, with the reporting taking more time away from care (Lloyd et al, 2014). The Ontario Staffing Study (Ontario, 2020, p 3) lists excessive documentation as one of the working conditions that must be addressed, along with low remuneration, part-time employment, and physical, mental and emotional risk. Although the high number of deaths in Ontario nursing homes during the COVID-19 pandemic pushed the government to promise a gradual increase in hours of care for residents and some improvement in staff pay, other working conditions are not being addressed.

In all three countries, women account for more than four out of five workers. A significant proportion of the workers are racialised, and this is particularly the case with the small but growing number of men. The preponderance of women and of those from racialised groups reflects assumptions that the skills required in the work are limited, as are the employment opportunities available to immigrants.

In sum, low funding, low staffing levels and low continuity, resulting from both high turnover and low rates of full-time employment, mean that there are significant gaps in care left to be filled by unpaid labour.

Inside nursing homes

The physical structure and location of nursing homes reflect and influence the assumptions about care at the same time as they have an impact on paid and unpaid care.

Resident rooms in Sweden and Norway are bigger and more private than in Ontario, and nursing homes tend to be smaller. A typical Swedish care home consists of 40 to 50 apartments in units of 8 to 12 residents, usually with a dining room and living room for each unit. Seventy per cent of residents have cognitive impairment, with about half of them accommodated in specialised dementia units (Stranz and Szebehely, 2018). Apartments are usually 30 to 40 square metres in size, almost all with a private bathroom and a kitchenette. Spouses are allowed to move in together, even if only one of them needs care. Except for the bed, residents are expected to bring their own furniture. These places are intended to be homelike and to meet both the social and the physical needs of residents. The combination of small units and both private and communal spaces, along with an increased focus on individualised care, have made residential care in Sweden more attractive than home care (Szebehely, 2017).

Norwegian nursing homes are like Swedish homes in size and housing standard. Almost all residents have a private room, and 90 per cent also have a private bathroom, although rooms are smaller than in Sweden and usually do not have private cooking facilities (Swedish Agency for Health and Care Services, 2021). The high proportion of RNs reflects a stronger focus on medical care than on social activities (Ågotnes et al, 2017).

Ontario legislation declares homes should provide 'a safe, comfortable, home-like environment' that supports 'a high quality of life for all residents' (Marrocco et al, 2021, p 32). However, many Ontario nursing homes look like hospitals. Units of 32 rooms are common, with long hallways and nursing stations. About 60 per cent of homes have more than 96 residents. Subsidies are available only for 'basic' rooms, which can accommodate as many as four people. And reflecting concerns that the extra fees charged for these amenities would restrict access, the number of private rooms with a bathroom is limited. New standards call for a maximum of two in basic rooms. Private rooms must be at least 12.1 square metres and other rooms must provide at least 11 square metres of space for each person (Ontario, 2015). A bed is provided but residents may bring their own furniture to fit into the small spaces. There are central dining and recreation areas, with size varying from home to home. Most homes have outdoor spaces, although access may be restricted to those who are accompanied. As in Scandinavia, most residents have some cognitive impairment and some are accommodated in specialised units (Marrocco et al, 2021, p 41).

All Ontario nursing homes are required to have a residents' council to support residents' participation in the home's decision-making and to provide educational opportunities. Family councils to advise the home leadership and to make recommendations for improvement are allowed but not required. In Ontario, secondary school students must complete 40 hours of volunteer work to graduate, and some of them volunteer in nursing homes. Community organisations also do volunteer work, providing a wide range of activities and services.

In sum, Swedish homes offer the most homelike spaces while Ontario's homes are the least homelike and their structure supports a more complex division of labour.

Implications for unpaid work in nursing homes

In all three jurisdictions, access to care is based on need rather than ability to pay. However, as Chapter 2 shows, the failure to provide enough beds to meet demand and the strict criteria for admission create significant unpaid work for applicants, their families and their friends in different ways in

Sweden and Ontario, reflecting the different conditions described in the previous section. This is a process made more complex by the lack of clear guidelines and attention to working conditions for the unpaid work of both staff and families. It thus raises important questions about recognising and supporting families, about access and about communications.

The next two chapters focus on particular kinds of unpaid work done within care homes. Chapter 3 sets out the range of body work, a type of work that is often not recognised and that is supported by unpaid work in often unrecognised ways. It compares practices and conditions in Sweden and Ontario, showing that supporting residents' autonomy, including their sexual expression, usually demands more rather than less paid staff time. Lower staffing levels and less emphasis on autonomy can therefore mean less self-care on the part of residents.

Approaches to care and their implications for social activities and social relations are explored in Chapter 4. The priority given to medical care and to easily measured tasks, combined with a more rigid division of labour, especially in Ontario, puts the emphasis on survival, leaving the social and relational side of living to be provided by unpaid workers. Although Chapter 4 explores the social activities and social relations through data from Ontario, that analysis is carried out jointly by a Norwegian and a Canadian, illustrating how our 'fresh eyes' approach allows a comparative way of seeing that draws out the implications of context for this essential work.

The next chapters take a different angle, analysing who does what kinds of unpaid work. The section begins with the unpaid work of residents. This labour has been largely invisible in the research on nursing homes and is seldom considered in policy and practice, even though as Chapter 5 shows, the work is profoundly shaped by both, with residents negotiating their care within specific contexts.

Chapter 6 turns to a form of labour that has become more visible with COVID; namely the unpaid work of families. What this chapter does though, that is different from other reports on such labour, is to look at the conditions under which this work is carried out, demonstrating the significance of approaching family participation as labour.

Chapter 7 takes up the question of how staff view this unpaid labour by families, another rarely explored issue, and one, as the chapter shows, that is quite differently shaped by conditions in the different countries. The changing working conditions for staff have an impact on their perspectives on the unpaid work of family and friends. Chapter 7 explains that while staff in Sweden, Norway and Canada all have mainly positive relationships with unpaid workers, in Ontario, families do more work to fill the care gap, undertaking tasks that are elsewhere done by paid staff. By contrast, in Sweden and Norway, the work of family and friends is primarily understood as that of social visitors and carriers of knowledge. Nevertheless, in all three countries staff experience tensions with families, and some of these tensions are about work.

The following two chapters take up questions of how unpaid work is structured in specific ways by location, connections and the broader context. Including all those who do unpaid work in the three countries, Chapter 8 analyses the ways rural and urban contexts influence unpaid work, showing how geographical and social mechanisms shape unpaid work differently in each of those contexts. Chapter 9 demonstrates the importance of integrating with the community outside the home, showing that communities can be brought together in ways that both support and alleviate pressures on unpaid workers. It explores the ways integration can create opportunities for residents to provide their own care, and for families as well as friends and volunteers to participate actively and imaginatively in the nursing home.

The final chapter explains why it is important to understand these unpaid activities as work. Funding, ideas about rights, the numbers and mix of staff, the extent to which they are employed full or part time by the home, along with the division of labour, all shape unpaid work. So do the time devoted to care and the approach to care. Locating the unpaid work and specific examples of that work within the multiple layers of policies, work and workers and capturing the complexity of relations among them, we contribute to our understanding of that work and of how we can support it in promising ways through changing policies, conditions and practices. All the chapters demonstrate that there is no fixed line between these different forms of labour and that there is no universal amount of unpaid work required to ensure care. Rather there are flexible boundaries between paid and unpaid work, a flexibility reflecting different normative frames, structural pressures, policies and practices. There are choices to be made.

References

Ågotnes, G., Jacobsen, F.F. and Barken, R. (2017) A Norwegian view on Canadian long-term residential care, *Journal of Canadian Studies*, 50(2): 491–98.

Ågotnes, G., Jacobsen, F.F. and Szebehely, M. (2019) The growth of the for-profit nursing home sector in Norway and Sweden: Driving forces and resistance, in P. Armstrong and H. Armstrong (eds) *The Privatization of Care: The Case of Nursing Homes*, Routledge.

Anttonen, A. (2002) Universalism and social policy: A Nordic-feminist revaluation, *Nordic Journal of Feminist and Gender Research*, 10(2): 71–80.

Armstrong, P. (2013) Puzzling skills, Special Issue 50th Anniversary of the *Canadian Review of Sociology*, 53(3): 256–83.

Armstrong, P. and Armstrong, H. (1990) *Theorizing Women's Work*, Garamond.

Armstrong, P. and Armstrong, H. (2016) *About Canada: Health Care*, Fernwood.

Armstrong, P. and Lowndes, R. (eds) (2018) *Creative Teamwork: Developing Rapid, Site-switching Ethnography*, Oxford University Press.

Armstrong, P., Armstrong, H. and Kehoe-McLeod, K. (2016) The threats of privatization to security in long-term residential care, *Ageing International*, 41(1): 99–116.

Armstrong, P., Banerjee, A., Szebehely, M., Armstrong, H., Daly, T. and Lafrance, S. (2009) *They Deserve Better: The Long-term Care Experience in Canada and Scandinavia*, Canadian Centre for Policy Alternatives.

Baines, D., Cunningham, I. and Shields, J. (2017) Filling the gaps: Unpaid and precarious work in the non-profit social services, *Critical Social Policy*, 37(4): 625–45.

Barken, R. and Armstrong, P. (2017) Skills of workers in long-term residential care: Exploring complexities, challenges, and opportunities, *Ageing International*, 43(1):110–22.

Bourgault, S. and Robinson, F. (eds) (2019) Resisting hierarchies through relationality in the ethics of care, *International Journal of Care and Caring*, 4(1): 11–23.

Canadian Institute for Health Information (CIHI) (2021) 'Long-term care homes in Canada: How many and who owns them?' Available from: https://www.cihi.ca/en/long-term-care-homes-in-canada-how-many-and-who-owns-them#:~:text=Ontario%20has%20a%20total%20of,not%2Dfor%2Dprofit%20organizations

Daly, T. and Szebehely, M. (2012) Unheard voices, unmapped terrain: Care work in long-term residential care for older people in Canada and Sweden, *International Journal of Social Welfare*, 21(2): 139–48.

Drange, I. and Vabø, M. (2021) A cross-sectional study of sustainable employment in Nordic eldercare, *Nordic Journal of Working Life Studies*, 11(7): 03–24.

Elstad, J. I. and Vabø, M. (2021) Lack of recognition at the societal level heightens turnover considerations among Nordic eldercare workers: A quantitative analysis of survey data, *BMC Health Services Research*, 21: 747.

Esping-Andersen, G. (1990) *The Three Worlds of Welfare Capitalism*, Princeton University Press.

Harrington, C., Choiniere, J., Goldmann, M., Jacobsen, F., Lloyd, L., McGregor, M., Stamatopoulos, V. and Szebehely, M. (2012). Nursing home staffing standards and staffing levels in six countries, *Journal of Nursing Scholarship*, 44(1): 88–98.

Harrington C., Dellefield, M.E., Halifax, E., Fleming, M.E. and Bakerjian, D. (2020) Appropriate nurse staffing levels for U.S. nursing homes, *Health Service Insights*, 13, doi: 10.1177/1178632920934785

Home Care Ontario (nd) 'Home care', Available from: https://www.homecareontario.ca/home-care-services/facts-figures/home-care

Kröger, T. (2003) Universalism in social care for older people in Finland – Weak and still getting weaker, *Nordisk Sosialt Arbeid*, 23(1): 30–34.

Land, H. and Rose, H. (1985) Compulsory altruism for some or an altruistic society for all?, in P. Bean, J. Ferris and D. Whynes (eds) *In Defence of Welfare*, Tavistock, pp 74–96.

Leira, A. (1994) Concepts of caring: Loving, thinking and doing, *Social Services Review*, 68(2): 185–201.

Lloyd, L., Banerjee, A., Harrington, C., Jacobsen, F. and Szebehely, M. 2014) "It is a scandal!": Comparing the causes and consequences of nursing home media scandals in five countries, *International Journal of Sociology and Social Policy*, 34(1/2): 2–18.

Luxton, M. (1980) *More than a labour of love: Three generations of women's work in the home*, Women's Press.

Marrocco, F.N., Coke, A. and Kitts, J. (2021) *Ontario's long-term Care*, COVID-19 Commission, Final Report, Available from: http://www.ltccommission-commissionsld.ca/report/pdf/20210623_LTCC_AODA_EN.pdf

National Board of Health and Welfare (Sweden) (2019) *Enhetsundersökningen om äldreomsorg och kommunal hälso- och sjukvård, 2019* [Survey on elderly care and municipal health care, 2019], Socialstyrelsen.

National Board of Health and Welfare (Sweden) (2022) *Statistics on Care and Services for Elderly and People with Impairments – Management Form 2021*, Socialstyrelsen.

Naylor, C.D. (1986) *Private Practice, Public Payment: Canadian Medicine and the Politics of Health Insurance, 1911–1966*, McGill-Queen's University Press.

Organisation for Economic Co-operation and Development (OECD) (2021) *Health at a Glance 2021*, Available from: https://doi.org/10.1787/ae3016b9-en

Ontario (2015) *Long-term Care Design Manual*, Available from: https://health.gov.on.ca/en/public/programs/ltc/docs/home_design_manual.pdf

Ontario (2020) 'Long term care staffing study', Available from: https://www.ontario.ca/page/long-term-care-staffing-study

Smith, D.E. (1987) *The Everyday World as Problematic: A Feminist Sociology*, Northeastern University Press.

Statistics Norway (2022) *Health and Care Institutions, Beds and Rooms by Type and Ownership*, Available from: https://www.ssb.no/en/helse/helsetjenester/statistikk/sjukeheimar-heimetenester-og-andre-omsorgstenester

Strandell, R. (2020) Care workers under pressure – A comparison of the work situation in Swedish home care between 2005 and 2015, *Health and Social Care in the Community*, 28(1): 137–47.

Stranz, A. and Szebehely, M. (2018) Organizational trends impacting on everyday realities: The case of Swedish eldercare, in K. Christensen and D. Pilling (eds) *The Routledge Handbook of Social Care Work Around the World*, Routledge.

Struthers, J. (2017) Home, hotel, hospital, hospice: Conflicting images of long-term residential care in Ontario, Canada, in S. Chivers and U. Kriebernegg (eds) *Care Home Stories: Aging, Disability, and Long-Term Residential Care*, Transcript Verlag, pp 283–302.

Swedish Agency for Health and Care Services (2021) *Den nordiska äldreomsorgen* [Nordic eldercare services], Vård- och omsorgsanalys.

Szebehely, M. (2017) Residential care for older people: Are there lessons to be learned from Sweden? *Journal of Canadian Studies*, 50(2): 499–507.

Szebehely, M. (2020) *Internationella erfarenheter av covid-19 i äldreboenden* [International perspectives on COVID-19 in care homes], Report for the Swedish Corona Commission, Available at: https://coronakommissionen.com/publikationer/delbetankande-1/

Szebehely, M. and Meagher, G. (2018) Nordic eldercare – Weak universalism becoming weaker?, *Journal of European Social Policy*, 28: 294–308.

Thompson, E.P. (1978) *The Poverty of Theory and Other Essays*, Merlin Press.

Van Aerschot, L., Mathew Puthenparambil, J., Olakivi, A. and Kröger, T. (2022) Psychophysical burden and lack of support: Reasons for care workers' intentions to leave their work in the Nordic countries, *International Journal of Social Welfare*, 31(3): 333–46.

Yakerson, A. (2019). Home care in Ontario: Perspectives on equity, *International Journal of Health Services,* 49(2): 260–72.

2

Accessing nursing home care: family members' unpaid care work in Ontario and Sweden

Petra Ulmanen, Ruth Lowndes and Jacqueline Choiniere

In this chapter, we show how state policies and the structural features of formal care systems in Sweden and Ontario, Canada, shape family members' unpaid care work for relatives in the lead-up to admission to a nursing home. This unpaid work includes the navigation and advocacy work required to seek, apply for and enter nursing home care. We also show how the entry of their relatives to nursing home care changes family members' unpaid care work in these two jurisdictions.

Sweden and Canada represent two social policy approaches to long-term care: a universal social democratic approach in Sweden, with a comparatively generous provision of tax-funded care services for all social groups (see Chapter 1), and a more selective liberal approach in Canada, with less generous public funding and one that requires residents to pay extra for private rooms and some additional services, meaning that an individual's financial situation affects the quality of care they receive (MacDonald, 2015). A higher proportion of older people receive home care or nursing home care in Sweden than in Canada, and staffing levels are also higher in Sweden (see Chapter 1). Both countries have, however, witnessed a rationing in long-term care funding, homes and services, but in different ways.

For over three decades, long-term care has been rationed in Sweden. Since 2000, the number of nursing home beds has declined by 30 per cent, informed by a strong 'aging in place' policy. Home-care services have not, however, received the resources necessary to meet the increased care needs in the community, and family members' unpaid care work has increased (Ulmanen and Szebehely, 2015; Schön and Heap, 2018). Today, 44 per cent of municipalities report a shortage of nursing home beds (NBHBP, 2021). With this steep decline, older people enter nursing homes later, are frailer, and tend to die sooner after entry (Schön et al, 2016), half of them within 18 months of admission (NBHW, 2020, p 107). Increasing standardisation and fragmentation of home care and home-care work leaves more clients with short visits from different care workers (see Chapter 1). Continuity of care and care work are disrupted, with limited worker discretion to meet clients' increasingly complex needs (Strandell, 2020), which may contribute to the fact that nursing homes are the preferred place to live for frail older people in Sweden (see Chapter 1).

In Canada, restructuring informed by neoliberalism has been shifting more care into people's homes, with a focus on 'aging in place', and nursing home care coverage has declined since the 2000s. Today, Ontario has lower nursing home care coverage than the Canadian average (see Chapter 1) and an extreme shortage of beds, with waiting times averaging 143 days (Canadian Health Coalition, 2018). The Ontario government's policy approach of Aging at Home and Home First, touted as ensuring enhanced patient–centred care and greater efficiency, has in fact led to reduced access to publicly funded home care (Armstrong and Armstrong, 2010; Grigorovich, 2020), leaving Ontarians with significant unmet home-care needs (Turcotte, 2014). Care rationing resulting from competitive bidding, where multiple providers submit offers to provide services, along with home-care funding cuts, negatively affects clients, families and providers (Armstrong, 2007; Grigorovich, 2020).

Previous research in both jurisdictions suggests that family members with extensive care responsibilities experience great stress leading up to the admission of their relative to a nursing home. As their relative's health deteriorates, care responsibilities and emotional challenges increase. After the move, family members' care work often changes and feelings of relief may be mixed with guilt, while responsibilities continue (Høgsnes et al, 2014; Høgsnes et al, 2016; Hainstock et al, 2017; Konietzny et al, 2018). Gaining access to nursing home care involves considerable unpaid work in terms of navigation and advocacy. Indeed, a 'structural burden' has been identified as arising from 'managing complex interactions with the fragmented structures of formal health and social care systems' (Taylor and Quesnel-Vallée, 2017, p 20). Funk and her colleagues point out that the 'structural features of formal care systems influence the amount, difficulty, and complexity of what carers do as they interface with those systems' (Funk et al, 2019, p 426). In this chapter we explore the impact of care systems on the unpaid care work of families.

Nursing home care systems in Ontario and Sweden

In 2015, the Canadian Medical Association reported that 88 per cent of Canadians surveyed wanted improved access to nursing home care (Ipsos Public Affairs, 2015). In Ontario, Home and Community Care, operating within 14 Local Health Integration Networks, assesses and manages nursing home admission and eligibility for home-care services (MHLTC, 2018). The delay in accessing nursing home care is considerable: the waiting list in February 2019 was 34,834 people for one of the 77,257 long-stay beds (OLTCA, 2019). Before being added to a waiting list, prospective residents must meet the criteria of the Method for Assigning Priority Levels. Given the shortage of beds, only people with high or very high needs are admitted to nursing home care (OLTCA, 2022). Although eligible clients can list up to five choices, they must take the first bed available in any of the chosen homes, or their application is cancelled, and they cannot reapply for 12 weeks (Government of Ontario, 2020). Furthermore, they have only 24 hours to consent to take a bed when one becomes available (OLTCA, 2022), and five days to move in (Government of Ontario, 2020), which adds to the stress. In an Ontario study, families reported 'chronic worry and burden', '[a] sense of lack of control' and 'perceived pushing, pressure, and punishment from the health care system' during the process of deciding on, applying for and transitioning their relative into nursing home care (Konietzny et al, 2018, p 464). Another Ontario study revealed the considerable physical, mental, social and financial costs for families of delayed admission (Um et al, 2020).

Sweden has a highly decentralised long-term care system, in which 290 municipalities in the country are responsible for financing and providing services. At the national level, the Social Services Act governing long-term care does not provide detailed regulations or specific rights. The design and execution of the law are the responsibility of municipalities, with care managers mandated to make decisions, including assessing and managing admission into nursing homes (Dunér and Nordström, 2006). Each municipality makes its own rules regarding how many homes eligible clients can apply to, how many days they have to take up a bed, and the outcome of declining a bed.

Although the national law states that individual needs should determine access to care, the assessment guidelines of many municipalities have become more restrictive with budgetary constraints (Dunér and Nordström, 2006; NBHW, 2011, p 162). The law requires that a person deemed eligible for nursing home care be admitted within three months, but waiting times have increased (NBHW, 2020, p 97). The combination of budgetary restrictions, bed shortages and the three-month requirement provides strong incentives for municipalities to reject applications rather than risk a fine for making eligible people wait too long. As a result, clients wait longer before their nursing home application is granted, and this kind of waiting time is not included in statistics.

Interviews with 33 family members with relatives in three Ontario and two Swedish nursing homes (located in different municipalities) form the basis of this analysis. In Ontario, 10 women and 2 men were interviewed, and in Sweden, 13 women and 8 men. We explore jurisdictional differences according to four themes: Trying to Manage at Home, Trigger Points, Navigating the System, and The Change After the Move.

Trying to manage at home

In both Ontario and Sweden, family members were very engaged in caring for their relative before the decision was made that they would move to a nursing home. Especially in Ontario, family members took on an excessive amount of unpaid work, including worrying about their relative, to provide for all of their relative's care needs so that they could keep them at home as long as possible. The wife of an Ontario resident described her constant fear that her disabled husband would leave the house without her noticing: "So he had Parkinson's. His mobility was very poor, but he didn't seem to know that his mobility was that poor. So he would take off with his walker. He would hitchhike. He would do whatever. He would usually do this when I was in the bathtub."

In both jurisdictions, we heard about families' struggles with inadequate home-care services. Family members' unpaid work encompassed all aspects of care, including personal and emotional care, ensuring medications were taken, arranging appointments and accompanying their relatives to them. Through it all, worry about their loved one's safety was constant.

Ontario family members often provided care with little or no outside help, reflecting the difficulties they had in accessing home care. Although their relatives received home care several times a day, most Swedish family members considered it insufficient to ensure safe, acceptable care. They complained that visits were too short and involved many different home-care workers, who were often late and pressed for time. A son explains why the needs of his 89-year-old mother, who had dementia, were not met by home care, even though care workers visited her five times a day:

'She couldn't plan and organise it and she couldn't get any help from them ... she was simply too ill. [There] was no extra help ... with things [she needed], which you might say was the idea [behind home care]. ... They were there 15 minutes, quickly warmed up the food [and asked], "Is there anything we can do here?" But there was no time [for her] to go to the lavatory and even less [for her] to sit down and eat properly. ... The system is simply worthless. It's only because it's cheaper for the taxpayers [that] they force it upon the residents, and it sounds good, "live at home". Why, it's pure neglect!'

Our Ontario participants told us that home-care services were not always readily available and that they did not always provide the quality desired. Only 3 of our 12 participants had home care, which worked well for the one who had the same personal support worker for four years; but the others expressed concerns. They told us about reduced hours, like this wife in Ontario: "It's so logical to me that it's so much cheaper for this province, country, whatever, to keep somebody at home than it is to put them wherever, OK. Why is providing adequate formal support such a problem?" Those without any outside formal services shared their struggles with us. One had hired private nursing care and had friends help to give medication, two were in private pay retirement residences before entering nursing homes, and yet another was a retired nurse who oversaw most of her husband's rehabilitation after his stroke herself.

Unlike in Ontario, no family member in Sweden told us about care managers cutting down on home-care hours without this having been requested by the care recipient. Most interviewees whose relative had home care twice a day or less were spouses. They refrained from applying for more home care in spite of the need, because they did not want several different people entering their home, or did not wish to wait around for them, not knowing when they would come. Instead, they wanted more privacy and to be in control of their own home. This was the case for a wife in Sweden, whose 86-year-old husband had home care twice a day and respite care every second week. When his needs increased, she requested a nursing home place, but the care manager wanted her to accept more home care instead:

'All the time, it was more home care, more home care, more home care, and I thought it was quite difficult because I had close friends who had had home care. They could get home care five times a day, but then [they had to] be home all the time to open the door. I mean, what should I do? … To let a lot of strangers go in and out of the apartment and I'm not at home myself, that does not appeal to me at all. So, it was quite enough with the home care we had in the morning and … the evening, [because] then the same persons came [each time].'

With some help from her adult children with re-applying, she finally succeeded in getting a nursing home place for her husband.

Most Swedish adult children interviewed had parents who were receiving home care several times a day, and the adult children were advocating for improved services, but with very limited success. As they were not living with their parent, they sometimes found it hard to determine how home care worked, which increased their worries. They did not know if they could trust either what home-care staff told them, or, because of their memory difficulties, what their parents said.

Trigger points

In both jurisdictions, people struggled with increasingly challenging circumstances as their relative became frailer and their condition worsened.

Many used the words "unsafe" and "intolerable" to describe their relative's situation at home. They told us about frequent acute hospital admissions, which were making them realise that their relative could no longer manage at home and needed nursing home care. A common trigger point, a pivotal event demonstrating that nursing home care was necessary, was a fall at home, which often resulted in a fracture.

In both countries, family members described how care professionals assisted in the decision to move their relative into a nursing home. An Ontario wife shared the following: "I got some help to look after him, but it became increasingly clear that it was less and less manageable … that I couldn't look after him. He wandered out. He wouldn't take his medication. It was just – I couldn't, couldn't really handle it."

When asked if she was waking up in the middle of the night worrying about him, she responded: "Oh of course, because I didn't – I couldn't trust him. He would go out. We have stairs going down and you know he would go out on the street. That's why [name of doctor] said to me, 'You can't manage'. … Which was true. I could not."

Navigating the system

The Ontario families who had positive experiences during their attempts to secure a nursing home bed were also those whose relatives were considered to be in a crisis situation. These individuals all reported not having to wait, and being "bumped up". A husband describes how he struggled with bathing his wife at home:

'I tried bathing her in the bath, but she was too heavy, and … she wouldn't sit down, wouldn't stand up. And so then I'd have her take showers, but she resisted, [with me] ending up almost in fist fights with my wife of 50 years. [Laughter] At least once I put her in the shower with her clothes on.'

He was encouraged to put his name on a list and the situation was eventually deemed a crisis, which resulted in him securing a bed quickly. However, others explained that much time was spent waiting and not knowing when their relatives would be offered a bed.

Advocacy was often required when needs increased. An Ontario wife described such a situation:

'I called this organisation, LHIN, and I think I had about four different people. … There was no continuity and … I have to start from scratch [each time] … and it became obvious that he needed to be placed and I had people come in to help me with [spouse]. And one day case manager number five is sitting there because she wanted me to sign some paper. ... [Spouse] is trying to take the furniture apart. He's got a walker because when he's got this boot on kicking things, and she's – out of the corner of her eye, she's kind of watching this and she finally can't stand it and she says, "Well I see you're busy!" She said, "I'll let you go". I said, "No, no, no, listen to me. You're gonna sit here and watch what goes on here". I said, "No, no, no, no. You need to, to see what I'm dealing with for 12 hours a day and you need to get my [spouse] into a home". She scurried out of there so fast, she didn't know what – so that was experience number one.'

Many Swedish family members had to advocate for an a nursing home place too, also experiencing a lack of continuity because several different care managers were handling their case. Family members in both countries had limited knowledge of the rules and regulations regarding assessments and admissions, which was an obstacle when they were navigating the nursing home care system. While Ontario family members got stuck on long waiting lists after having been deemed as qualifying for nursing home care, in Sweden people commonly got stuck in the actual process of applying for placement, either because their applications were rejected, or because they did not have the care recipient's consent so the municipality could accept the application. (This consent is not required in Ontario.) Once the Swedish care manager accepted an application, the process of choosing and moving into a nursing home was generally quite quick, taking between a few weeks and a few months.

A rejection made some Swedish family members wait until their relative's needs got more extensive before applying again, while others chose a more offensive strategy and re-applied almost immediately and repeatedly. Some even appealed against the rejection in court. Three adult sons with higher education used the offensive strategy.

Even in cases of severe cognitive decline, Swedish care recipients have to give their consent to moving into a nursing home (or at least not oppose it) for the application to be granted by the municipality. If the prospective recipients are able to oppose such a move, no custodian or administrator can override that. This is, however, a grey area, both legally and in practice (Ryrstedt, 2014). This way of getting stuck was experienced by a daughter whose 88-year-old mother had been diagnosed with dementia 10 years earlier but had declined nursing home care when her daughter and son had applied for it:

'Home care did unpaid extra hours at my mother's and we were there practically every day, me and my brother, and wore ourselves out. Well, that's why it worked, sort of, but at the end it didn't even work. Then the police picked her up and called us ... and the people on the street called (she had the telephone numbers on her walker) and said, "Hi there's a lady here who ..." So, I went out looking for her, I don't know how many times. And then the police, they got involved of course. ... And at the end, of course, she heated things in the microwave oven and she tried to make a fire so she almost set the house on fire.'

The daughter and her brother made another nursing home care application. It was not granted. Later on, when their mother was admitted to hospital due to a back injury requiring the use of a wheelchair, a care manager was able to convince her to not oppose admission to a nursing home. Their nursing home application was finally granted.

A new care manager cleared away the last obstacle by asking the mother in a way that she would not oppose.

In both countries, family members normally visited a number of nursing homes in order to determine suitability, while also considering their relative's wishes. They were, however, unanimous in wanting their relative in a nursing home within close proximity. We also heard about the anxiety family members experienced when faced with the pressure to accept an offer within a very short period of time – 24 hours in Ontario and around three days in Sweden. One Ontario daughter lamented:

'[W]e had booked a flight down to [another province] to help ... my former sister-in-law and to visit a granddaughter who'd just got to university. And we got off the plane and we got into our car in the parking lot at the airport and I picked up my phone and I looked and it said, "Your mom is being offered a bed at [nursing home] and you have 24 hours to decide". ... And so, I was overwhelmed with that. I just sat and cried in the car and I didn't know what to do.'

Required to make such a major decision in a short time created much stress for family members. Moreover, once the decision was made to accept the offer, in Ontario families only had five days to get their relative moved in, while in Sweden families had around a week. Family members had a lot of unpaid work to do during this time, from preparing the relative emotionally for the move to making all the necessary decisions and practical preparations.

The change after the move

Most families in both countries were happy with the home their relative was in, and for the majority it was their first choice. A few had moved their relative from another home because they were not satisfied with it or because they wanted their relative close by to be able to visit more often.

Many family members also saw their relative as less lonely than they were at home because they were now within a community (see Chapter 9).

For Ontario family members, the unpaid care work continued after admission. We heard from those who visited their relative every day and arranged for (or provided) haircuts, did the relative's laundry, performed daily care activities such as shaving, and took their relatives on outings and to all medical appointments. When family members did not give direct care, they shared the stress of ensuring that care was provided. A sister described the unpaid care work along with the advocacy efforts:

> 'I do worry about him when I see him unshaven. I gave everybody a lecture on the floor. I said, "There are enough indignities in this disease, so please humour me". I have his clothes all organised. So all they have to do is pick it up. "So humour me and make sure his hair is brushed. He's shaven. Blah blah blah". So yes. And that's why I insist on going there every day. … He's the first thing in my mind when I wake up … and usually when I go to bed.'

Yet another wife shared with us her feelings of guilt, and worry, and told us about her ongoing unpaid work of arranging for family and friends to visit when she could not be there.

In contrast, most Swedish family members described the nursing home admission as a turning point and a great relief. Safety and continuity of care increased with staff present 24/7, and the family's responsibility for care was willingly relinquished. Families explained that their relative was not left alone for long periods of time any more and if something happened, they received help quickly, which eased the families' worries. Although most saw the need for some improvements, they generally trusted the staff and saw little need for advocacy.

The son who previously described his mother's intolerable situation at home explained the difference after nursing home admission:

> 'Well, you cannot compare. Except, there are several things that all of a sudden work without really asking. The hygiene – now mother is clean and is wearing clean clothes and receives help with visiting the lavatory and with diapers and all that. So, the hygiene works automatically, immediately. The other thing that works automatically is that she no longer eats too little – she gets food and meals at regular hours. … So, everything is better. And in addition, the safety. Then you know there is supervision. When she falls out of bed or something, a nurse is there. They are used to this type … get to the hospital or call the doctor if it is needed. So that's totally safe, you know.'

Most Swedish family members visited the nursing home at least once a week, and some visited every day. They continued taking their relative to medical appointments, providing emotional support and monitoring the care provided, and some tidied up their relative's apartment, but they seldom provided personal care (see Chapter 8).

Structural features shaping unpaid care work

Our findings illustrate the numerous levels and types of unpaid work taken on by family members for their relatives in the lead-up to their admission to nursing homes and during the process of being admitted, and the changes that take place after admission. They also signal the differences between Sweden and Ontario in the nature of this unpaid work, which is related to the ways in which care is organised in these jurisdictions.

Interviews from Ontario and Sweden indicate similarities and differences among families trying to manage at home (the first of our four themes). In both jurisdictions, families struggle to access adequate home-care support, albeit from systems that differ in significant ways. Ontario family members shared stories of the intense stress of trying to manage individuals with increasingly complex needs at home, which was ultimately down to an overall rationing of care. On the other hand, Swedish family members recounted the inadequacies of a home-care system that readily offered additional short, standardised visits by carers, which instead of providing the quality of care needed, resulted in more fragmented care. Families in both jurisdictions described increased stress and unpaid care work due to receiving too few, or too many inadequate, visits. This clearly contradicts the literature citing the importance of relational-based continuity of care (Peckham et al, 2021). The result was an increase in stress and unpaid care work for families.

Another difference between the two jurisdictions relates to families' opinions about nursing home care. In Ontario, there seemed to be an aversion to nursing home care, a finding supported by other Ontario research showing that families viewed nursing home care "as a last resort, [to be avoided] as long as possible" (Um et al, 2020, p 10). Swedish families were more positive about nursing home care, with our interviews indicating they were more likely to request it and that there was greater disappointment when their request was denied, and more home care offered instead, which may be an effect of care rationing of another kind. While the steep decline in the number of Swedish nursing home beds resulted in an increasing number of older people with extensive needs living at home, home-care rationing meant an increased number of short visits by different care workers. Both ways of rationing imply a clear deviation from the policy aim of universalism, which entails accessible, affordable and attractive long-term care (Vabø and

Szebehely, 2012). Instead, in Sweden, nursing home careis becoming less accessible and home care less attractive.

Our interviews also highlight similarities in both countries regarding the trigger points (Theme 2) that alerted families and care providers to things becoming too difficult for their relatives to remain at home. Yet they suggest a greater level of stress on the part of Ontario families as they come to the realisation that their relatives require more intensive care and that they can no longer provide it. Comments such as "[I] couldn't really handle it" and attempts at assisting with a relative's personal care "ending up almost in fist fights" are reflective of that stress; and they support other research identifying such a decision as an emotional crisis, and one imbued with guilt (Um et al, 2020). While both jurisdictions report having an Aging in Place policy direction, our interviews suggest stronger support for home care on the part of families in Ontario. We did not witness the same level of guilt or preference for home care among the Swedish families interviewed, probably because they have experienced the inability of home care to meet their relatives' complex needs. With the Swedish welfare state promising to take primary responsibility for meeting care needs but failing to meet home-care needs, the nursing home option probably becomes more attractive and less imbued with guilt. In addition, the higher staffing levels in Swedish nursing homes make them a better option than in Canada.

Our interviews suggest some similarities in navigating the system (Theme 3). Families in both countries reported a lack of knowledge about the access process, and described the complicated nature of making the right decision. They shared how their stress increased when faced with many different individuals guiding them through the process, while their relatives' needs grew increasingly complex. Further, the short time allowed to accept or reject a nursing home bed created tensions. In Ontario, the pressure to accept the first available nursing home bed placed families in a very difficult situation. When the decision was made, the short time provided to move in added to the stress in both jurisdictions.

In Sweden, the assessments and decisions around applications are decentralised and less formal, compared to the centralised and formal application processes in Ontario. While there is lack of choice in both countries, it is of a different variety. Waiting times are much longer in Ontario and family members are more likely to get stuck *after* being deemed eligible, suffering physical and mental consequences as a result (Um et al, 2020). In Sweden, families get during stuck *in* the application process because of rejections and having to re-apply, and in cases where they do not get consent from the relative to apply. While advocacy is often required throughout the process of accessing nursing home care in Ontario, in Sweden advocacy is most needed up to the point that the application is accepted; after that it generally works smoothly and quickly. The need for advocacy, however, conflicts with the Swedish policy commitment to universalism, as it favours those families with the greatest resources in terms of higher education, absence of cognitive decline, and resourceful family members, such as the sons with higher education who re-applied the highest number of times and even appealed against rejections of applications in court.

The similarities and differences in the experiences of family members in the two jurisdictions continue after the move (Theme 4) into nursing homes, with a higher level of concern on the part of Ontario families. This is reflected in their continued strong engagement in their relatives' care, their active participation in that care, and their ongoing need to advocate for better-quality care. They were stressed by the need to make sure care was provided and by the guilt they felt when they were unable to visit. In contrast, nursing home admission was a significant relief for Swedish families. They were pleased with the continuity of care, which was now available 24/7, and expressed relief over having to provide much less unpaid work, including navigation and advocacy. The persistent worrying about their relatives' unsafe situation at home was no longer necessary either. Swedish family members expressed more trust in the staff and few expressed the need for ongoing advocacy. This may reflect the higher staffing levels in Swedish nursing homes, combined with a growing disappointment with home care.

As our research indicates, neoliberal reforms in both jurisdictions are evident in reduced access to nursing home care and in the rationing of care. They are manifested in similar, new public management approaches in both countries, yet with varying implications. In Sweden reforms are reflected in increasing numbers of short, focused home-care visits, which delay nursing home admissions (Strandell, 2020). In Ontario, competitive bidding, in addition to home-care funding cuts, rations home care, in spite of declining nursing home carecoverage (Daly, 2007; Grigorovich, 2020). There are different implications of these responses in the two countries. In Sweden, family members criticise the short, focused home-care visits, expressing concern about the loss and devaluing of relational aspects of care and the failure to consider differences in individual needs. At the same time, the family's unpaid advocacy and management work increases, as nursing home care becomes more difficult to access. The Ontario interviews reflect a higher level of daily care work at home, and more stress and worry as well as more advocacy work in the face of resistance to requests for more home care. There is also a continuation of care work responsibilities after the nursing home admission, in contrast to Sweden, which may reflect greater access and higher staffing levels in Sweden.

The reaction to nursing home admission offers a clear contrast. While Ontario interviews revealed aversion to and guilt about the move into a nursing home, those with respondents in Sweden indicated families were much more supportive of nursing home care and even advocated for it. As

Armstrong and Banerjee (2009) have argued, nursing home admission in Canada tends to be viewed as a failure of the individual to stay healthy and a failure of the family to fulfil its responsibilities, reflecting a strong emphasis on individual responsibility, unlike the support for collective responsibility that characterises the social democratic foundations in Sweden.

References

Armstrong, P. (2007) Relocating care: Homecare in Ontario, in M. Morrow, O. Hankivsky and C. Varcoe (eds) *Women's Health in Canada: Critical Perspectives on Theory and Policy*, University of Toronto Press, pp 528–53.

Armstrong, P. and Armstrong, H. (2010) *Wasting Away: The Undermining of Canadian Health Care*, Oxford University Press.

Armstrong, P. with Banerjee, A. (2009) Challenging questions: Designing long-term facility care with women in mind, in P. Armstrong, M. Boscoe, B. Clow, K. Grant, M. Haworth-Brockman, B. Jackson, A. Pederson, M. Seeley and J. Springer (eds) *A Place to Call Home: Long-term Care in Canada*, Fernwood Publishing, pp 10–28.

Canadian Health Coalition (2018) 'Ensuring quality care for all seniors', Policy Brief, Available from: http://www.healthcoalition.ca/wp-content/uploads/2018/11/Seniors-care-policy-paper-.pdf

Daly, T. (2007) Out of place: Mediating health and social care in Ontario's long-term care sector, *Canadian Journal on Aging*, 26(S1): 63–75.

Dunér, A. and Nordström, M. (2006) The discretion and power of street level bureaucrats: An example from Swedish municipal eldercare, *European Journal of Social Work*, 9(4): 425–44, https://doi.org/10.1080/13691450600958486

Funk, L.M., Dansereau, L. and Novek, S. (2019) Carers as system navigators: Exploring sources, processes and outcomes of structural burden, *The Gerontologist*, 59(3): 426–35, https://doi.org/10.1093/geront/gnx175

Government of Ontario (2020) *Long-term Care Overview*, Queen's Printer, Available from: https://www.ontario.ca/page/about-long-term-care

Grigoriovich, A. (2020) Satisfaction not guaranteed: Broadening the discourse on quality improvement in the home care system, in E. Mykhalovskiy, J. Choiniere, P. Armstrong and H. Armstrong (eds) *Health Matters: Evidence, Critical Social Science, and Health Care in Canada*, University of Toronto Press, pp 131–51.

Hainstock, T., Cloutier, D. and Penning, M. (2017) From home to 'home': Mapping the caregiver journey in the transition from home care into residential care, *Journal of Aging Studies*, 43: 32–9, https://doi.org/10.1016/j.jaging.2017.09.003

Høgsnes, L., Melin-Johansson, C., Norbergh, K.G. and Danielson, E. (2014) The existential life situations of spouses of persons with dementia before and after relocating to a nursing home, *Aging & Mental Health*, 18: 152–60, https://doi.org/10.1080/13607863.2013.818100

Høgsnes, L., Norbergh, K.G., Danielson, E. and Melin-Johansson, C. (2016) The shift in existential life situations of adult children to parents with dementia relocated to nursing homes, *The Open Nursing Journal*, 10: 122–30, https://doi.org/10.2174/1874434601610010122

Ipsos Public Affairs (2015) *Canadian Medical Association 2015 National Report Card: Canadian Views on a National Seniors' Health Care Strategy*, Ipsos Public Affairs, Available from: https://www.ipsos.com/sites/default/files/publicat ion/2015-08/6959-report.pdf

Konietzny, C., Kaasalainen, S., Dal-Bello Haas, V., Merla, C., Te, A., DiSante, E., Kalfleish L. and Hadjistavropoulos, T. (2018) Muscled by the system: Informal caregivers' experiences of transitioning an older adult into long-term care, *Canadian Journal on Aging*, 37(4): 464–73, https://doi.org/10.1017/S0714980818000429

MacDonald, M. (2015) Regulating individual charges for long-term residential care in Canada, *Studies in Political Economy*, 95(1): 83–114, https://doi.org/10.1080/19187033.2015.11674947

Ministry of Health and Long-term Care (MHLTC) (2018) 'Local Health Integrated Network home and community care services', Available from: https://www.health.gov.on.ca/en/common/system/services/lhin/facts.aspx

National Board of Health and Welfare (NBHW, Sweden) (2011) *Hälso- och sjukvård och socialtjänst: Lägesrapport 2011* [Health and social care: Progress report 2011], Available from: https://www.socialstyrelsen.se/globalassets/sharepoint-dokument/artikelkatalog/ovrigt/2011-2-1.pdf

National Board of Health and Welfare (NBHW, Sweden) (2020) *Vård och omsorg om äldre. Lägesrapport 2020* [Health and social care for older people. Progress report 2020], Available from: https://www.socialstyrelsen.se/globalassets/sharepoint-dokument/artikelkatalog/ovrigt/2020-3-6603.pdf

National Board of Housing, Building and Planning (NBHBP, Sweden) (2021) 'Underskottet på särskilda boendeformer har minskat betydligt' [The shortage of nursing homes has declined considerably], Available from: https://www.boverket.se/sv/samhallsplanering/bostadsmarknad/olika-grupper/aldre/sarskilda/

Ontario Long Term Care Association (OLTCA) (2019) 'Shaping the future of long-term care. About long-term care in Ontario: Facts and figures', Available from: https://www.oltca.com/oltca/OLTCA/Public/LongT ermCare/FactsFigures.aspx

OLTCA (2022) 'Long-term care services and the application process', Available from: https://www.oltca.com/oltca/OLTCA/Public/LongT ermCare/Services.aspx

Peckham, A., Williams, P., Denton, M., Berta, W. and Kuluski, K. (2021) "It's more than just needing money": The value of supporting networks of care, *Journal of Aging & Social Policy*, 33: 201–21, https://doi.org/10.1080/08959420.2019.1685357

Ryrstedt, E. (2014) Får jag inte bestämma något själv? En studie av kvarstående beslutanderätt hos dementa äldre [Can't I decide anything by myself? A study of the remaining right to make decisions among older people with dementia], *Socialvetenskaplig tidskrift*, 21: 3–4, https://doi.org/10.3384/SVT.2014.21.3-4.2409

Schön, P. and Heap, J. (2018) *ESPN Thematic Report on Challenges in Long-term Care. Sweden 2018*, EU Network of Independent Experts on Social Inclusion, European Commission, Available from: https://ec.europa.eu/social/BlobServlet?docId=19870&langId=en

Schön, P., Lagergren, M. and Kåreholt, I. (2016) Rapid decrease in length of stay in institutional care for older people in Sweden between 2006 and 2012, *Health & Social Care in the Community*, 24: 631–38, https://doi.org/10.1111/hsc.12237

Strandell, R. (2020) Care workers under pressure: A comparison of the work situation in Swedish home care 2005 and 2015, *Health and Social Care in the Community*, 28(1): 137–47, https://doi.org/10.1111/hsc.12848

Taylor, M.G. and Quesnel-Vallee, A. (2017) The structural burden of caregiving: Shared challenges in the United States and Canada, *The Gerontologist*, 57(1): 19–25, https://doi.org/10.1093/geront/gnw102

Turcotte, M. (2014) 'Canadians with Unmet Homecare Needs', Statistics Canada, Available from: www.statcan.gc.ca/pub/75-006-x/2014001/article/14042-eng.pdf

Ulmanen, P. and Szebehely, M. (2015) From the state to the family or to the market? Consequences of reduced residential eldercare in Sweden, *International Journal of Social Welfare*, 24(1): 81–92, https://doi.org/10.1111/ijsw.12108

Um, S., Sathiyamoorthy, T. and Roche, B. (2020) *The Cost of Waiting for Long-term Care: Findings From a Qualitative Study*, Wellesley Institute, Available from: https://www.wellesleyinstitute.com/wp-content/uploads/2021/01/The-Cost-of-Waiting-for-LTC-Findings-from-a-Qualitative-Study.pdf

Vabø, M. and Szebehely, M. (2012) A caring state for all older people, in A. Anttonen, L. Häikiö and K. Stefánsson (eds) *Welfare State, Universalism and Diversity*, Edward Elgar, pp 121–143.

3

Body-work-that-isn't: supporting nursing home residents' autonomy in self-care and sexual expression

Susan Braedley

Taking care of bodies – body work – is central to nursing home care. Typically described as the 'direct, hands-on activities, handling, assessing and manipulating bodies' that 'involves both a knowledge of the materiality of the body and an awareness of the personhood that is present in that body' (Twigg et al, 2011b), it encompasses the physical work involved in cleaning, dressing, feeding and toileting people who are unable to perform these tasks on their own, and the interpersonal interactions that facilitate these tasks.

Many residents are active in caring for their own bodies, continuing to dress, shower, feed themselves and more, depending on their capabilities. In the nursing home context where resident bodily care is an institutional responsibility, this resident self-care is a variety of 'unpaid work', contributing to the overall work required to maintain the nursing home population.

It is rational to surmise that if some residents do this bodily care for themselves, workers will have less to do. If body work is defined narrowly, this is correct. But supporting a resident's autonomy in self-care can take more, not less, staff time, creativity, coordination and energy than just doing the body work for the resident. This work is what I call 'body-work-that-isn't': the work involved in promoting and supporting resident autonomy in bodily self-care and sexual expression. I argue that this work is important to a resident's well-being and dignity but regularly goes uncounted and undetected in job descriptions, policy and organisational workflows and processes.

Typically, nursing home body work is understood to include tasks involving specific workers who perform them, the residents who passively endure or enjoy this service, and the interpersonal connections that facilitate this work (Twigg et al, 2011a, 2011b). Although staff do most body work in nursing homes, families and volunteers contribute too. And family members often express strong opinions about how 'their' resident is cared for, influencing how body work is performed by staff (Chang and Yu, 2013). But at the centre of these concerns is the resident – a person working to maintain a sense of self, meaning and agency while experiencing frailty and disability. Although nursing home residents require 24/7 nursing support, many residents express their autonomy and sense of self through bodily self-care and sexual expression. Dressing, undressing, bathing, grooming oneself, going to the toilet and eating unassisted have significance beyond completing tasks of daily living. Across cultures, jurisdictions and social differences of gender, race, sexuality and class, this self-care is, for many residents, a marker of 'independence' and an important symbol of personhood. Bodily sexual expression in this context is another opportunity to express and experience selfhood, offering sensory pleasure and possibilities for intimacy and connection. It is also resistance to stereotypical depictions of older people as asexual, undesirable and undesiring (Heidari, 2016).

Nursing home body work and self-care activities have different implications than the same activities performed in other contexts. For some, body work is an indulgence, a luxury and a status symbol. Those who are able-bodied and with sufficient means can have someone else wash and style their hair, give them a manicure, facial or shave, or provide sex work, signalling agency and the means to choose and direct service providers.

For those with disabilities, body work can be an existential requirement, not a luxury. Disability activists and advocates have taken an individual rights approach to ensuring body work for those whose lives rely upon it. A key demand has been to provide those with disabilities with the power to choose and direct both this work and those who provide it (Shakespeare, 2000). Most congregate forms of care are resisted or rejected by these movements.

Congregate living and caring offers a very different approach to care and to body work. In publicly funded and regulated congregate long-term care environments, the available care is a shared social resource, not an individual service. In these settings, the right to receive care is not understood as the right to choose and direct care, or as a quantity of care delivered in a particular time frame. Instead, it is the right to a share of the available care. If residents are to share care equitably on the basis of need, direct care staff must have sufficient autonomy to allot their work time to observing and responding to resident needs, determining care priorities as needs change.

For residents and their families, congregate care requires the continual negotiation of a tension between resident autonomy and institutional rules and responsibilities. Institutional rules vary, but often include rigid, externally determined times for meals, bedtimes and activities. Residents and staff often have little say in determining how the day's activities will proceed. Workers continually navigate the blurry boundaries created by this tension with awareness of their often conflicting responsibilities to residents, funders, families, employers, and other workers. In our research, concerns about institutional reputation were noted in every site study, suggesting another variety of responsibility.

Given these conditions, residents' options for choice and control over their care are limited, both individually and collectively. Unlike resident representation in university residences or retirement homes, such representation in nursing homes is limited by abilities and energies, and by organisational failures to establish mechanisms for meaningful resident representation. Further, residents' frailties limit their opportunities to spend time away from the nursing home. Most residents, once admitted to care, spend almost all their days and nights inside the walls of their institution, and have no choice about it.

This limited resident autonomy, choice and control play out in the relational dynamics associated with body work. If residents' personhood is to be fully considered while tensions between resident autonomy and institutional responsibility are negotiated, body work must have a flexible boundary, where workers have discretion to support residents' autonomy to look after their own bodies in ways residents choose. This is body-work-that-isn't. Rather than direct hands-on body care, this work supports residents' involvement in caring for their own bodies and desires.

This body-work-that-isn't includes supporting resident autonomy in sexual expression. Residents' frailty and disability, combined with the congregate care environment, remove any possibility of privacy about sexual activity, and prevent residents from accessing supplies for sexual expression, such as pornography and toys. Workers and family members are often involved in restraining and addressing residents' inappropriate sexual behaviours, including towards themselves (Braedley et al, 2017; Daly and Braedley, 2017; Grigorovich and Kontos, 2020; Grigorovich, et al, 2021). But workers and family members are also able to support or limit residents' agentic sexual expression.

I draw on data collected in team ethnographies conducted at public and non-profit nursing homes in Ontario, Canada and Sweden,[1] to explore how resident autonomy in bodily self-care and sexual expression can be supported. This analysis reveals the time, complexity and coordination required to provide body-work-that-isn't. This work is not outlined in most nursing home job descriptions and goes unrecorded in workload measures.

The data analysis began with the aim of understanding and comparing how body work was performed in these contexts. Interview transcripts, fieldnotes, institutional forms and processes were coded. As the findings about supporting self-care and sexual expression emerged, representative vignettes were developed from the data using two criteria: they should highlight issues that had emerged repeatedly in our ethnographies, across contexts; and they should illustrate situations that demonstrated a promising practice. These criteria offer an alternative to tendencies in long-term care research that pathologise resident and worker distress (Dupuis et al, 2012; Joseph, 2017) and/or depict congregate care as irretrievably problematic Herron et al, 2021).

In this article, three vignettes are presented. These vignettes show how managers and workers understood, documented, discussed and addressed bodily self-care situations within specific nursing homes in our studies. They also indicate how the tensions between resident autonomy and institutional responsibilities were negotiated. Most importantly, the vignettes show how different conditions of work and care allowed resident autonomy and choices to be supported, suggesting promising practices and opportunities for change.

An Ontario vignette: Joe's socks, negotiating regulations and staffing constraints

For Joe, moving to a nursing home was a defeat. As he told it, "I never thought this would happen to me". Every morning, he dressed himself, displaying self-efficacy, maintaining his self-worth and dignity, and resisting self-judgments of helplessness and failure. Dressing himself allowed Joe to say, "I don't know why I am here".

But socks had become a challenge. Unable to bend over, Joe sat on his bed and lifted a foot off the ground while he took a sock in one hand, leaned forward and hooked his toes into the top of the sock. Grabbing the sock with both hands, Joe slowly slid off the low bed, sinking to the floor with leg extended, hands on the sock. Success! The sock was on.

Minutes later, a care aide found Joe sitting on floor, struggling to hook his other sock onto his toes. "What happened, Joe? Are you hurt?" "Not a bit!" said Joe. "Well, I have to get the nurse to check you out, so don't move."

Together, the nurse and care aide helped Joe stand and shift onto the bed. Although Joe was not happy about it, the nurse examined him, finding no injuries. Later, the nurse recorded Joe's sock-finagling in the resident data system as a 'fall', defined as 'an unintentional change in position coming to rest on the ground' (CIHI, 2012).

"Joe, we can help you get dressed in the morning. You just wait, and the care aide will give you a hand. We don't want you hurt!"

But Joe was not persuaded. Care aides and nurses recorded Joe's falls on many more mornings. At the end of the month, the Nurse Manager did her regular review of the resident data, saw the fall pattern, asked about it and learned about Joe's sock technique. The nurses stopped counting Joe's sock slides as falls; his change in elevation was clearly intentional.

Luckily, in Joe's nursing home – a non-profit organisation that had supplemental funding beyond the government funding allocation – Joe was supported to continue to dress himself. The nursing staff lowered his bed to reduce his slide, watched for injuries when they helped Joe to shower, and checked on him while he was dressing. The Nurse Manager kept an eye on Joe's developing dementia and its impact on his cognition or balance.

When Joe's son visited from another city, Joe told him, "I dress myself every day!"

Analysis of Joe's case

As Joe's case reveals, nursing home conditions can encourage and support or discourage and prevent resident's self-care. But no matter what conditions exist, staff are continually involved in negotiating the tension between resident autonomy and institutional responsibility. In this situation, support for Joe's sock routine did not emerge as a question of how to best support resident autonomy in self-care or to prevent injury. It emerged as an issue of accurate reporting and risk to the nursing home's reputation.

Joe's 'falls' went almost unnoticed at the unit level.[2] Problems with staffing were partly responsible for this oversight. Only a few personal support workers (PSWs) and nurses worked consistently in Joe's resident unit. Although this large nursing home had lower staff turnover and fewer part-time and temporary care workers than most nursing homes in Ontario, it experienced constant staff scheduling challenges and shortages. On a typical morning, four PSWs and a registered practical nurse provided care to 32 residents, overseen by a registered nurse who supported up to four units. During our ethnography, PSWs were working 'short', and so the ratio of staff to residents was lower than that. Although consistent unit staffing was an aim, staff shortages and turnover led to many temporary rotations and re-assignments, with only a few workers working regularly in the same unit. The workers did not always know each other well enough to coordinate the work easily, and only some workers knew the residents well enough to notice patterns of behaviour. Acting in these short-staffed conditions, PSWs and nurses worked rapidly to assist residents needing high levels of support and did not always check on the more independent residents. Finally, the unit staff's only regular opportunity to discuss resident care was at shift change, when they focused on acute resident health or behavioural issues, and not on intervention strategies or quality-of-care matters. Our research team noted few lags in nursing staff activity that would allow for such discussion. These conditions of work meant that the pattern of Joe's falls was easily missed at the unit level, potentially risking his self-care.

Unit nursing staff followed regulations and recorded Joe's 'falls', allowing the pattern to be noted by the Nurse Manager. The Nurse Manager became an investigator, speaking to Joe, PSWs and nurses to sort out the issue. She directed workers to stop recording Joe's routine as a fall and coordinated the team to support Joe's self-care.

Resident data are collected in this and other nursing homes in most Canadian provinces and internationally via the Resident Assessment Instrument/Minimum Data Set (RAI/MDS). This standardised assessment tool, instituted in 2010 in Ontario, is used by Canadian provincial and territorial government funders to assess the quality of care in nursing homes and to 'rationalize services and systems' (Armstrong et al, 2017). For example, Quality Ontario, the provincial health system monitoring agency, uses these data to publish nursing home fall rates as one metric in its quality assurance programme (Health Quality Ontario, 2023). They are also used to calculate resource allocations relative to resident acuity measures. The RAI/MDS focuses on medical risk and does not include data on resident autonomy or satisfaction (Daly et al, 2020), supporting a strong long-term care 'audit culture' (Banerjee, 2013; Banerjee and Armstrong, 2015) that prioritises data collection on residents over direct care to them. It is possible that this was a factor in Joe's case.

Once the Nurse Manager had intervened, workers supported Joe's autonomy in dressing. They helped him get up from the floor, rather than putting on his socks for him. This change meant a departure from the usual routine as well as staff coordination across shifts and professional hierarchies. For PSWs, supporting Joe to dress himself was more difficult and at least as time-consuming as dressing him. It required interpersonal skills, knowledge of Joe's ways and preferences, more physical effort, and, according to one worker, some self-talk to resist interpreting Joe's actions as an old man's stubborn behaviour that made extra work for an already taxed staff.

That this nursing home supported Joe's sock routine is not only a victory for Joe. It is a strike at the high degree of bio-medicalisation in Ontario nursing homes, which shapes responses to resident frailty via geriatrics rather than gerontology.[3] Such an approach means that medical risks, staff efficiency and home reputation are prioritised; dignity, choice, meaning, pleasure and relationships, while valuable, are often secondary.

In this home, despite structural barriers, creative, capable workers supported Joe by negotiating the tensions between resident autonomy and institutional responsibilities to provide body-work-that-isn't. They sorted out rules, priorities and reputational concerns, prioritising Joe's well-being. But it is also a precarious victory. Workers seldom have time to read all the notes in a file, and staff shortages and changes mean that tacit knowledge of resident choices is often lost in the process.

A Swedish vignette: Anna's shower, negotiating dementia, and time to problem-solve

Anna, a resident in a dementia-specific floor in a Swedish nursing home, had become anxious about showering. Showering had been Anna's preferred way to bathe, and she had participated actively in washing herself. Recently, she had become agitated and distressed about getting a shower and had stopped participating. Mostly non-verbal, Anna couldn't express reasons for her changed behaviour, but her cries and physical thrashing relayed her discomfort to the assistant nurses who supported her and who now dreaded struggling with Anna to get her washed.

The assistant nurses discussed the situation among themselves and other nursing staff at their regular hour-long 'reflection group' staff meeting. At this nursing home, staff were assigned permanently to specific areas of the home to work with a small team who cared for the same group of seven residents. On this dementia floor, regular paid time was set aside for staff to discuss care-related issues and solve problems connected with them. The team included two assistant nurses with specialised dementia care training, who supported fellow workers and educated and trained families and staff. One of these specialised assistant nurses facilitated the regular 'reflection group' meetings.

The team discussed Anna's situation. "We need to check with her doctor. Maybe medical issues are involved?"

"The only change in Anna that we know about is her eyesight – she isn't seeing nearly as well. Do you think that might be a factor?"

"Maybe. … The shower room walls and floor are almost the same colour. It might be difficult for her to distinguish them. That would be unsettling! And the white soap is on a white soap dish – she may not be able to see it now."

"We could try to put the soap on a coloured dish and get brightly coloured towels for her to use. Perhaps that might help?"

At the following team meeting, the assistant nurses gave the team an update. The doctor had adjusted Anna's medication, and she had become calmer and more "present", rather than anxious and hyperactive, during her shower. The coloured soap dish and towels seemed to support Anna to re-engage in soaping and drying herself, despite her sight limitations.

Analysis of Anna's case

For Anna, involvement in bodily care was a familiar activity that seemed to offer some sensual pleasure. Given her stage of dementia, it was impossible for staff to determine whether this involvement provided her with a sense of self-efficacy, but her "presence" and calm, combined with her efforts to wash and dry herself, signalled to the workers that Anna was enjoying her shower routine once again.

Problem identification in this case began when staff noticed Anna's avoidance and agitation as changes in behaviour signalling a change in her condition. The issue was not that Anna's dementia or blindness was advancing, nor that her health was at greater risk because she was less clean, nor that Anna required more support and was using more staff resources, nor that her family was complaining, although all these circumstances may have been involved. Instead, the issue was that Anna was more anxious and agitated, and less engaged in her bodily care. Staff wanted her to experience calm and pleasure, and to enjoy self-care.

Given Anna's non-verbal status and dementia, to notice her behaviour change as a pattern related to showering, and not just a 'bad day' or another episodic anomaly, is contingent on staffing conditions. It requires a staffing complement assigned to the same group of residents, employed for sufficient hours per week, with significant work time directly spent with residents, and with sufficient training to know how to observe, assess and interact. Only these circumstances allow staff to acquire sufficient knowledge of the behaviour, moods and preferences of the frail and disabled residents to distinguish patterns of behaviour, indications of illness or distress, and shifts in, for example, visual acuity.

In this Swedish home, the nursing-staff-to-resident ratio was relatively high compared to ratios in Ontario and many other jurisdictions, with one worker for every three residents in the dementia unit where Anna lived. This home's overall worker-to-resident ratio was slightly higher than the 3.3-residents-per-worker average in Sweden's relatively generous welfare regime, and almost double the ratio in Joe's Ontario nursing home. This staffing was stable, and turnover was low. Overall, the staff were very well trained, and some workers at the home had taken specialised dementia training.[4]

Further, to support personalised care, residents and their familial caregivers filled out an extensive form, called *Dokumentet om mig* or 'Document about me'. The document required residents to describe their life and preferences, including bodily care, hairstyle, skin care, nails, showering and washing, toileting, makeup, shaving and clothing, as well as their fears and daily routines. The document outlined the nursing home's commitment to ensuring that workers reviewed this information and that workers would ask residents what they wanted to do in caring for themselves, letting them do what they could, and supporting them when they needed help. While Ontario nursing homes use similar documents to record resident preferences, the level of detailed attention to resident autonomy and choice in this Swedish example stood out in our international research.

Embedded in Swedish social care legislation are commitments to 'dignified life and well-being' in nursing homes (Socialtjanstlag, 2001, quoted in Nilsson et al, 2018, p 50). Specifications for personalised care are provided by the Swedish National Board of Health and Welfare (SOSFS, 2012), which states that 'an individual's self-determination and participation must be strengthened' (Nilsson et al, 2018, p 50). While Sweden's nursing home sector is experiencing marketisation (Meagher and Szebehely, 2013; Harrington et al, 2017) and deteriorating working conditions (Stranz and Szebehely, 2017), the commitments made in these policies were put into operation in some nursing homes. These policies created opportunities to negotiate the tensions between institutional responsibility and resident autonomy via relatively generous funding for staffing. The case of Anna's shower illustrates this point.

Principles, knowledge and nice promises are insufficient to support self-care, however. Regular reflection meetings and trained dementia care nursing staff allowed this Swedish team to put knowledge into action. Discussing how to approach particular care issues and reporting on successes and failures allowed them to learn, develop skills and provide consistent support to resident autonomy and involvement in bodily self-care.

Comparing Joe's situation with Anna's, it is apparent that both residents were supported in their bodily self-care as a result of actions taken by skilled, compassionate staff. In Ontario, the outcome was facilitated through a system of risk management and data collection and required a thorough nurse manager to 'discover' what was happening. But the direct care staff who did the work were not engaged in problem-solving or getting to know Joe well. There were no processes that could ensure this approach to Joe's care was maintained if staff changed. In Sweden, a well-trained, consistent and relatively generous staffing complement supported both Anna and the workers. Her positive outcome was facilitated by designated, institutionally set staff time for creativity and consultation. In the Swedish case, it didn't take a manager to notice and investigate. Rather, the workers closest to Anna were able to arrange both medical consultation and alterations in the physical environment to support Anna's self-care.

Bodily care includes sexual expression

The sexual expression of residents is not usually considered when discussing nursing home bodily care, but in the context of frailty and disability, sexual activity, like most other activities, requires support. In considering body-work-that-isn't, this analysis includes staff involvement to support or discourage resident autonomy in bodily sexual expression.

While old age tends to reduce the frequency of sexual activity, it does not reduce sexual interest (Taylor and Gosney, 2011). For residents, sexual expression offers both pleasure and intimacy. Sexual expression may offer residents some continuity in self-concept, and the chance to resist ageist ideas of older people as asexual. It can offer pleasurable sensory stimulation and an opportunity to experience a familiar, welcome ritual. Some residents value sexual expression as important to their sense of self and enjoyment of life (Grigorovich et al, 2021). However, in the context of congregate care, privacy is not possible and the staff and family involved in care often discourage and constrain resident sexual expression. For those with dementia, sexual expression is often interpreted as sexual disinhibition – inappropriate behaviour to be managed through pharmaceuticals (Cipriani et al, 2016).

In our ethnographies, residents, staff and family members often raised issues related to sexual activity (Daly and Braedley, 2017). This vignette from Ontario reveals the issues involved in negotiating tensions between resident autonomy and institutional responsibilities regarding sexual expression, while showing the involvement of body-work-that-isn't.

An Ontario vignette: Elsbeth's sex life and negotiating consent

Experiencing late-stage dementia but still physically healthy, Elsbeth has lived at a 130-bed nursing home in a small Ontario town for three years. Slowly she has become non-verbal, showing little response to human interactions. Andrew, her husband of 60 years, recently moved into an adjacent unit of the nursing home and visited Elsbeth daily. Both staff and family believed that Elsbeth enjoyed Andrew's visits, as she was more animated afterwards.

During routine washing, PSWs noticed Elsbeth had developed a terrible rash in her pubic area. In discussing the situation among themselves and with other nursing staff, they deduced that the rash was a reaction to Andrew's use of hand sanitiser as a sexual lubricant. They discussed it with the Nurse Manager, who took it to the nursing home CEO.

For the CEO and Nurse Manager, this discovery raised concerns about Elsbeth's ability to provide sexual consent and, if her family complained, the possibility of a lawsuit. Further, under the law in Ontario, a person with power of attorney cannot consent to sex on behalf of a dependant. The Nurse Manager contacted the couple's daughter, Andrea, who had power of attorney for both parents, to explain the issue.

Andrea said, "Let me tell you about my mom. She used to come down in her negligée and she was always, 'Come on, Andrew, it's time for bed!' We as kids would be like, 'Ohhh nooo!' Right? … It was all a very important part of their life together".

The Nurse Manager responded, "I don't know how we are going to stop this. Your mom is not in distress and your dad is not showing sexual aggression in interactions with her or other residents, based on our assessment. But you cannot consent on her behalf. Maybe we could be pro-active?"

Andrea agreed to talk with her siblings and extended family. With their agreement, she brought in a safe sexual lubricant for her parents' use. The Nurse Manager took notes on her conversations with the family and recorded all actions taken in both residents' files. Informally, the CEO consulted a lawyer with expertise in elder abuse, capacity and consent, who reportedly indicated that the home had "done the right thing".

Elsbeth and Andrew carried on their sexual relationship, unaware but now well supported by the nursing home staff and their entire extended family. Their body-work-that-isn't supported Elsbeth's continued sexual expression with her husband.

Analysis of Elsbeth's case

Even marital sex requires body-work-that-isn't in nursing home life. In this case, Andrew and Elsbeth's sex life was supported by unit staff both before and after the rash raised issues for managers and family. It is important to note that this couple's sex life was not ignored by unit staff but rather was handled discreetly. Staff had noted Andrew's daily visits, which had left clothing and bedding in disarray, and Elsbeth's positive change in demeanour after these visits. They had communicated with staff in Andrew's home unit, who were able to confirm he was not sexually predatory with other residents. In the context of this medium-sized nursing home, with relatively stable staffing, few issues with staff shortages, and a positive team dynamic, communication and knowledge flowed along informal as well as formal channels. In this case, staff communication had quietly supported these residents' autonomy in sexual expression.

Because the rash was a medical concern, any pretence that staff did not know about Andrew and Elsbeth's sexual expression was precluded, and their discretion to support it quietly was removed. Ethical and legal issues emerged because of Elsbeth's dementia and the possibility that her sexual activity was not consensual.

The Manager and the couple's family were formally notified and took over problem-solving. If the Manager had decided to take a narrow view of consent, or if family members had prevaricated or objected, no doubt the outcome of this situation would have been different. While family members may not provide legal consent to sexual activity on behalf of a relative, they are able to prevent sexual activity, and Andrew might have been moved to another nursing home. In this case, both the nursing home management team and the family actively supported the couple's sexual expression.

Care was facilitated by the blurry boundaries between work and community life typical of small communities. Our team was told about residents who had taught workers at school, or who had lived in the same neighbourhood or belonged to the same faith community. Without romanticising small town existence, in this case, community connections supported trust between the institution and the family, facilitating body-work-that-isn't, and helping to contribute to conditions that allow workers to negotiate the tension between resident autonomy and institutional responsibilities.

Body-work-that-isn't: what matters?

Drawing divisions between nursing home body work, what nursing home workers do to support resident bodily self-care, and resident self-care is like drawing lines in custard. One minute the lines are clear, the next, they're gone. But that blurry boundary is necessary to a staff team's capacity to negotiate tensions between resident autonomy and institutional responsibilities. In each vignette, these tensions showed up differently but were negotiated in a way that offered a promising practice and positive outcome for the resident involved.

Common to each positive outcome were conditions that allowed staff to get to know the residents involved, assess their situation, negotiate constraints and problem-solve to support residents. These conditions varied, however, and different types of staff were involved in resident support in each case. In the Ontario examples, managers were important, owing to the reputational concerns arising from both cases and administrative imperatives to manage these risks. In Sweden, workers not only had more time to care than in Ontario, they also had discretion to raise concerns about care, and opportunities to learn more. But these conditions were not enough. Positive outcomes in this context relied on capable staff who knew the residents well and worked collaboratively to negotiate tensions in order to ensure resident autonomy and choice.

Time to care is central to these matters. It often takes a resident more time to do their own care than it takes a worker to do it, so if a resident needs a worker to support them, then workers are not able to move from resident to resident as quickly. Given the rigidities of many nursing home mealtimes and activity schedules, taking more time for dressing, washing and toileting can mean a resident is late or misses their meal, physiotherapy or activity. Given constraints and limits to nursing home staffing in many jurisdictions (Harrington et al, 2012; Jacobsen et al, 2018; Laxer et al, 2016), taking time to support a resident can increase strain on other workers, and undermine possibilities for strong team relationships.

Time is money in these situations. Body-work-that-isn't is a continual aspect of nursing home life, requiring staff time to not only stand by and work with residents, but also to negotiate rules and regulations, contact family and organise worker cooperation. It is not only staffing levels and assignments that are important to this often uncounted and unrecognised work. Jurisdictional and organisational policies that only allocate sufficient funding for minimum staffing levels and low wages produce conditions in which this work is impossible or seldom accomplished.

What matters to supporting resident autonomy in bodily self-care and sexual expression, then, is what has been pointed out repeatedly by many researchers. Congregate care for frail, disabled and dying people offers opportunities for collective living and reliable, competent shared care, with benefits for both residents and workers. But resident autonomy and involvement in their own care relies on workers and managers who have the time, the capacity and both the professional and the relational knowledge to negotiate tensions between resident needs and organisational responsibilities.

Notes

[1] Ethnographic material was drawn from Ontario and Swedish site studies from SSHRC-funded 'Changing Places: Unpaid Work in Residential Places' (PI: Pat Armstrong, York University), and Ontario site studies from CIHR-funded 'Seniors: Adding Life to Years' (PI: Janice Keefe, Mount Saint Vincent University).

[2] Nursing homes are divided into 'floors' or 'resident home areas', otherwise called units. A unit is a designated physical area of a nursing home that contains a number of resident 'beds'. In these studies, units ranged in size from seven to eleven beds in Sweden to 32 beds in Ontario.

[3] While gerontology takes a holistic approach to aging that includes physical, mental and social aspects, geriatrics is a medical specialty focused on the care and treatment of older persons. See Estes (2019, pp 38–39), for a discussion of biomedicalisation that indicates 'a preference for geriatrics over gerontology in the competitive science of aging and its practice and policy'.

[4] See www.silviahemmet.se for details on this dementia certification programme.

References

Armstrong, H., Daly, T. and Choiniere, J. (2017) Policies and practices: The case of RAI-MDS in Canadian long-term care homes, *Journal of Canadian Studies* 50(2): 348–67.

Banerjee, A. (2013) The regulatory trap: Reflections on the vicious cycle of regulation in Canadian residential care, in G. Meagher and M. Szebehely (eds) *Marketisation in Nordic Eldercare*, Stockholm University Department of Social Work, pp 203–16.

Banerjee, A. and Armstrong, P. (2015) Centring care: Explaining regulatory tensions in residential care for older persons, *Studies in Political Economy*, 95(1): 7–28.

Braedley, S., Owusu, P., Przednowek, A. and Armstrong, P. (2017) We're told, "suck it up": Long-term care workers' psychological health and safety, *Ageing International*: 1–19.

Canadian Institute for Health Information (CIHI) (2012) *Resident Assessment Instrument (RAI) MDS 2.0 User's Manual*, Canadian version.

Chang, S.-H. and Yu, C.-L. (2013) Perspective of family caregivers on self-care independence among older people living in long-term care facilities: A qualitative study, *International Journal of Nursing Studies*, 50(5): 657–63.

Cipriani, G., Ulivi, M., Danti, S., Lucetti, C. and Nuti, A. (2016) Sexual disinhibition and dementia, *Psychogeriatrics*, 16(2): 145–53.

Daly, T. and Braedley, S. (2017) Let's talk about sex … in long-term care, in P. Armstrong and T. Daly (eds) *Exercising Choice in Long-term Residential Care*, Canadian Centre for Policy Alternatives, pp 69–77.

Daly, T., Choiniere, J. and Armstrong, H. (2020) 4 Code work: RAI-MDS, measurement, quality, and work organization in long-term care facilities in Ontario, in E. Mykhalovskiy, J. Choiniere, P. Armstrong and H. Armstrong (eds) *Health Matters: Evidence, Critical Social Science, and Health Care in Canada*, University of Toronto Press, pp 75–91.

Dupuis, S.L., Wiersma E. and Loiselle L. (2012) Pathologizing behavior: Meanings of behaviors in dementia care, *Journal of Aging Studies*, 26(2): 162–73.

Estes, C.L. with DiCarlo, N.B. (2019) *Aging A-Z: Concepts Toward an Emancipatory Gerontology*, Routledge.

Grigorovich, A. and Kontos, P. (2020) Problematizing sexual harassment in residential long-term care: The need for a more ethical prevention strategy, *Canadian Journal on Aging / La Revue canadienne du vieillissement*, 39(1): 117–27.

Grigorovich, A., Kontos, P., Heesters, A., Martin, L. S., Gray, J. and Tamblyn Watts, L. (2022) Dementia and sexuality in long-term care: Incompatible bedfellows?. *Dementia*, 21(4), 1077–97.

Harrington, C., Choiniere, J., Goldmann, M., Jacobsen, F.F., Lloyd, L., McGregor, M., Stamatopoulos, V. and Szebehely, M. (2012) Nursing home staffing standards and staffing levels in six countries, *Journal of Nursing Scholarship*, 44(1): 88–98.

Harrington, C., Jacobsen, F.F., Panos, J., Pollock, A., Sutaria, S. and Szebehely, M. (2017) Marketization in long-term care: A cross-country comparison of large for-profit nursing home chains, *Health Services Insights*, 10. 1178632917710533.

Health Quality Ontario (2023) System Performance: Long-term Care Home Performance, Available from: https://www.hqontario.ca/System-Performance/Long-Term-Care-Home-Performance

Heidari, S. (2016) Sexuality and older people: A neglected issue, *Reproductive Health Matters*, 24: 1–5.

Herron, R., Kelly, C. and Aubrecht, K. (2021) A conversation about ageism: Time to deinstitutionalize long-term care?, *University of Toronto Quarterly* 90(2): 183–206.

Jacobsen, F. F., Day, S., Laxer, K., Lloyd, L., Goldmann, M., Szhebehely, M., and Rosenau, P. V. (2018). Job autonomy of long-term residential care assistive personnel: A six country comparison, *Ageing International*, 43(1): 4-19.

Joseph, A. (2017) Pathologizing distress: The colonial master's tools and mental health services for 'newcomers/immigrants', in. D. Baines (ed) *Doing Anti-Oppressive Practice: Social Justice Social Work*, Ferwood, pp 233–51.

Laxer, K., Jacobsen, F.F., Lloyd, L., Goldmann, M., Day, S., Choiniere, J. and Vaillancourt Rosenau, P. (2016) Comparing nursing home assistive personnel in five countries, *Ageing International*, 41(1): 62–78.

Meagher, G. and Szebehely, M. (2013) *Marketisation in Nordic Eldercare: A Research Report on Legislation, Oversight, Extent and Consequences*, Department of Social Work, Stockholm University.

Nilsson, M., Jönson, H., Carlstedt, E. and Harnett, T. (2018) Nursing homes with lifestyle profiles: Part of the marketisation of Swedish eldercare, *International Journal of Care and Caring*, 2(1): 49–63.

Socialtjänstlag (2001) Social Services Act, 2001:453, Available from: http:// www.riksdagen.se/sv/dokument-lagar/dokument/svensk-forfattningssaml ing/socialtjanstlag-2001453_sfs-2001-453

SOSFS (2012) Värdegrunden i socialtjänstens omsorg om äldre: Socialstyrelsens författningssamling, 2012:3, Stockholm: Wolters Kluwer, sfs-2001-453. Government Bill. 2001/01:80. *Ny socialtjänslag m.m.* [New Social Services Act].

Shakespeare, T. (2000) The social relations of care, in G. Lewis, S. Gerwitz and J. Clarke (eds) *Rethinking Social Policy*, SAGE, pp 52–65.

Stranz, A. and Szebehely, M. (2017) Organizational trends impacting on everyday realities: The case of Swedish eldercare, in Christensen, K. and Pilling, D. (eds) *The Routledge Handbook of Social Care Work Around the World*, Routledge, pp 45–57.

Taylor, A. and Gosney, M.A. (2011) Sexuality in older age: Essential considerations for healthcare professionals, *Age and Ageing*, 40(5) September 2011: 538–43, https://doi.org/10.1093/ageing/afr049

Twigg, J., Wolkowitz, C., Cohen, R.L. and Nettleton, S. (2011) Conceptualising body work in health and social care, *Sociology of Health & Illness*, 33(2): 171–88.

4

"They make the difference between survival and living": social activities and social relations in long-term residential care

James Struthers and Gudmund Ågotnes

Under Ontario's Long-term Care Homes Act 2007, care homes are required to operate so that residents 'may live with dignity and in security, safety and comfort and have their physical, psychological, social, spiritual and cultural needs adequately met' (Ferreira, 2021). This objective is juxtaposed to what research indicates is a growing sense of loneliness among aging cohorts, leading increasingly to the social isolation of seniors, which is associated with certain risk factors, including reduced health (Grenade and Boldy, 2008; Freedman and Nicolle, 2020). This social isolation is presented as both a societal issue, in local communities, and as a health risk in long-term residential care settings, warranting adaptive and responsive service provision (Smith, 2012). It is also an issue that needs further research (Van Regenmortel et al, 2016). There is a dearth of knowledge, for instance, about how to enhance social connection among aging cohorts (Suragarn et al, 2021).

Perhaps as a response, there has been a growing academic focus over the past decade on the key role of meaningful social activities in combatting loneliness and promoting the well-being of people in long-term residential care (Knight and Mellor, 2007; Harmer and Orel, 2008; Theurer et al, 2015; Smith et al, 2018; Ågotnes and Øye, 2018; Lowndes et al, 2020). An important theme in this literature is a shift in focus away from the formal recreational and therapeutic programming delivered by trained professionals in care homes towards the more informal, spontaneous and multi-faceted roles played by unpaid family members, volunteers and residents themselves (Barken et al, 2016; Ågotnes and Oye, 2018; Lowndes et al, 2020; Hande et al, 2021), and the various forms of work they participate in (see also Chapter 1).

In all this literature, the significance of unpaid work, particularly that performed by women family members and volunteers, looms large. As Hande et al (2021) argue, within the Canadian context of widespread staff shortages in nursing home care, and the growing frailty of the NH population, 'paid caregivers have little time to engage in interpersonal work and relational resident care. Unpaid informal caregivers (predominantly family) often struggle to "fill the gaps"' (p 2). The role and contribution of unpaid work is also highlighted and problematised in other jurisdictions (Kröger and Leinonen, 2012; Grootegoed et al, 2015; Ulmanen and Szebehely, 2015; Ågotnes et al, 2021). Here, a shift in responsibility from paid (private or public) service provision towards unpaid contributions, particularly those of family members, is seen in the context of neoliberal reforms and austerity measures representing, in some contexts, 'a withdrawal of the state'. Canadian patterns of understaffing are connected to wider international trends. While NH care differs between jurisdictions, with regards to the role of volunteer organisations, the composition of staff and residents and ownership status, responses to what Hande and colleagues describe as a pronounced deficit of 'interpersonal work' seem to be increasingly shared.

On the basis of 35 interviews, conducted between 2017 and 2019 with staff, family members, volunteers and residents in three long-term care homes in Ontario, Canada, we explore the tensions, the rewards and the unexpected outcomes of this unpaid work of informal caregiving. We concentrate on the particular kinds of skills, knowledge and experience family members and volunteers require, as well as the challenges they face, in their efforts to protect and enhance the social life of nursing home residents. We found five key areas to be particularly important:

- gaining knowledge of residents' past lives and interests;
- bringing the outside interests of family members, volunteers, and residents into long-term care homes;
- encouraging friendships with other residents, family members, staff, and volunteers;
- developing intergenerational initiatives that regularly bring children into long-term care sites;
- highlighting the role of family members and volunteers in getting residents outside of their rooms.

Gaining knowledge of residents' past lives and interests

Given the increasing frailty and cognitive decline of residents in nursing homes, staff rely heavily on family members to tell them what activities residents might want to be involved in. Staff, volunteers and family members sought to apply knowledge of residents' interests and preferences to their everyday life within the facilities, attempting to accommodate the needs of individuals and groups of residents when they were incapable of expressing them. One recreation facilitator said, "We often need family to help us. … To fill out their history, tell us what their passions are, what they did with their leisure time". These activities are vital to residents' overall quality of life. As the wife of a resident told us: "They make the difference between survival and living."

Family members and volunteers provide a critical link to this information and to finding ways to use it to enhance residents' quality of life. This theme emerged powerfully in our interviews. One key example was reanimating musical memories. A family member, for instance, stressed his role as an informal music therapist for his relative as well as for other residents:

'I got to a point of bringing my laptop, because Mom loves music. ... Her dad played violin, [and] they loved "Down East", Don Messer's music, so I play that and all kinds of other old stuff. ... So, the next week I went back, the PSW on the floor that I really like best came over to me and said, "That was really good that you played that music". She said, "The people were so happy afterwards". So I said, "If you want I'll come back every week and do it". "Wow, that would be great." So, I used to go there every week on Friday morning. I'd play music there. ... So, I started doing that, and one old guy didn't even know, he just came in the door ... just as I started playing 'The Green, Green Grass of Home', an old standard, and his eyes lit up. "That's my favourite song," and he said he hadn't heard it in 30 years, right ... and I had some women that literally would sit here so that they could hear it.' (Interview with son)

A daughter explained how important music was for her mother:

'At one point I thought Mom was starting to lose her memory more so than she is now, but I think maybe she's recovered a bit, and maybe it's because of the music. So, she's in a wheelchair and then she comes to listen to the music, or even this morning for exercise they want to put her wheels on a lock so she doesn't move around, and I said, no, no, no ... so if there's music she sits and she rocks with the music, taps her toes and all that stuff, and I know what's happening – it makes her feel happy. She remembers when she was younger, dancing with her sisters and all the people that we'd grown up with that played music, but it was local country people; they'd all come together at the local hall and they'd have a hall party basically. So, you have to stimulate the brain one way or another.'

Family members and volunteers also noted how learning about the past lives of residents could provide an opportunity to encourage them to take up similar activities while in care:

'The resident across from my dad's room, he was actually the brother of our paper man ... this fellow retired and his wife used to deliver our paper. Anyways, his brother ... moved in across, [and] he ended up being the paperboy on this unit. ... So he'd get the newspapers because about half a dozen people had subscriptions and his job every day was to go get the subscriptions and deliver them. ... So he had a job every day and it was helpful.' (Interview with volunteer and family council member)

Bringing outside interests into nursing homes

The particular interests, skills and passions of family members and volunteers were also brought into the homes, enriching the variety and scope of social activities and the quality of life on a daily basis. This theme was prominent in the interviews conducted in each of our three Ontario sites. In one home, a resident who had previously owned a restaurant was allowed to organise a special dinner for all the residents once a month. It was named after his old business:

'They've made it into a programme. Once a month, [first name of resident]'s Pantry, it's dinner night, and he drives it, and he helps them in the kitchen, and he makes the menu, and they, they have him totally involved in the programme. There's great pictures of him in the kitchen stirring. That's what it's all about. He's so proud. Like "Come to my restaurant one night a month". You know, sometimes you go, "What are you doing? You can't make them do that". We're not making anybody do anything. It's about what they want to do. It's about involving them.' (Interview with Director of Community Outreach)

Family members and volunteers in this home also brought vital workplace skills and experience from their current or previous lives to help improve the quality of life for residents:

'Having worked for the government and the education department, I strongly believe in policy. You have a policy, then you find out it's working or it's not working. If it's not working, let's analyse why, and let's find ways to fix it. So, the other team I'm working on is the quality improvement team. ... I can – in terms of my husband's care, I can rant and rail that this isn't right or that isn't right, but tell me what the policy is, and then I'll know where we have to give and where you have to give.' (Interview with family member)

Volunteers who were former nurses also found their former workplace skills transferred beneficially into their new roles. "I knew ... I had a lot to give from my knowledge of bedside nursing", a volunteer at a smaller rural home told us. "If you have a resident that might be somewhat agitated … I don't get upset by that."

Artistic skills also emerged as key volunteer contributions in this home. "There was a very strong former art teacher … who was a real mover and shaker here. … She started the photography club, she started the art shows," two volunteers told us. Inspired by her work, they were now doing publicity to get members of the outside community to come into the home to see the art on display. At this same home, volunteers played a critical role in advocating over two years for the installation of a Wi-Fi service that residents and family members could access. "Even if people have dementia they still love to hear the voice of the people they love," we were told by two volunteers. This achievement would prove crucial during the subsequent COVID-19 pandemic, when family members were prevented from visiting residents for months at a time.

In this home, as in the others, family visitors helped greatly by bringing in music and pets.

> '[A]lmost everyone can come to the music programme, right? Or if there's children involved, so they really like that, or dog therapy. Obviously all these facilities have dogs come through and we really do encourage families if they have a dog that's well behaved – they're welcome in the unit. So they also bring their pets and that's great for the resident.' (Interview with Resident Special Program Coordinator)

Family members also made themselves available to grow food at the home. The same Resident Special Program Coordinator told us, "[T]his year we grew tomatoes. This year a family member came forth and said, 'I'd love to contribute. I'll bring the soil and plant the tomatoes and then we care for them, and we grew peppers and cucumbers".

Residents could put their gardening skills to use for the benefit of the entire home. As one told us, "Yeah, I help out a lot with the gardening. … [D]uring the summer time we grow tomatoes, peppers … I kept a bunch of seeds from the peppers we grew last year so I started growing them … and tomatoes and stuff".

Encouraging friendships

Bringing the past into the present and conveying skills and interests from the outside to the inside helped to create social bonds between residents, family members, staff and volunteers. A common refrain from family members who spent hours each day in homes visiting their relatives is how often they were mistaken for staff by other residents. "I mean, some think I work here, but [laugh] I'm here so often," said one. The rural location of this home allowed for a closer personal connection between family members and staff. As the daughter of one resident told us, "I'm from a small town myself and actually ... I was getting a lot of feedback about how ... staff members here knew a lot of the residents. They had been, you know, their cousins, grandmother or the neighbour down the street".

A family member from a more urban home stressed how critical she felt it was for her to develop strong personal bonds with all the staff involved in her husband's care. "I now end up a lot talking to the PSWs. I know everybody. I know the laundry. I know the cleaning lady. I have made it my business to know everyone by name. And some of the PSWs, we've bonded because they're with him for eight hours." She also made sure their work was recognised. "Well, I treat the staff very well at Christmas. I know I have about ten, ten people that last Christmas I gave them $25 each ... if it means in any way, shape or form that somehow my [spouse's name] is gonna get better care, that's fine by me." Another family member appreciated the importance of the emotional support staff had done for her recently deceased husband. "Even though he had given them such a run for their money, the staff said he was one of their 'all-time favourite residents'."

Family members in one of our two urban homes acknowledged the unpaid work of staff who gave up a Saturday to help organise a barbecue; who crocheted shawls for residents in their spare time to help keep them warm; who dropped in, after their shifts had ended, to visit a resident undergoing emergency care; or who took the time to set up equipment in the activities room so that a resident could do her own ironing: "That's a huge thing for my mother for her to be able to do that" (Interview with daughter).

A wife commented on the importance of a cafeteria worker taking the time to learn about her husband's life so she could help him eat. "If she wants him to come into the dining room, she'll say, 'Mr [last name], there's some students here that want to see you'. Because he was a principal ... and – and this is the cafeteria lady that figured this out. And I couldn't figure this out." A husband stressed how vital his own regular visits were to letting staff know they couldn't just "park" his wife in front of a TV. "I'm there every day, so I mean they know. It's not that they're, that I'm keeping an eye on them. I don't think they have that kind of opinion. But they know I'm there and I appreciate it and so they know I want her not left in her room as much as they have to."

As far as informal care work was concerned, bonds were important not only between families and staff, but also between families and other residents, and different families. Friendships formed among residents, family visitors and volunteers in homes emerged as a key resource for providing additional unpaid support, care and work. One family member told us she brought in food sometimes for other residents, offered them compliments and tried to make connections with them, in the hope that other visitors would reciprocate during her absence. "I always think, I wish, I hope somebody's thinking of [my brother] when I'm not here." A volunteer in a different home made a similar argument about the power of friendships forged with residents as an unanticipated reward for getting involved:

'Some of them do want to chat with us and we do get to know them and make friendships. Like [name of other volunteer] has been away lately and we haven't been here for a few weeks and when we came in today, we were just greeted like long-lost friends. The ones that are aware were very happy to see us.' (Interview with volunteer)

A recreation facilitator made the same point:

'I didn't mention it but support – families – will come in regularly, they'll see another resident and maybe just start chatting with them and then next time they come they'll say, "Hello [name]!" and they'll visit [name] for a while as well as their loved one.'

Two volunteers who took the initiative to form a committee to bring the art of local artists into their facility told us that one sure sign of a good nursing home was when family members continued to stay involved as volunteers, as they both had, after their loved ones had died. They felt a shared sense of "ownership" in the home through their continuing activities in it. A family member in a different home echoed the theme. Participating in social activities for other residents, she told us, "makes you feel like you're part of a family". She planned to stay on as a volunteer, even after her mother died: "If my mum were to pass I would stay on family council and probably at that point I would do more [as a] volunteer." A resident stressed the importance of her roommate's daughter in her life: "[She] comes and brings me gifts for my birthday and Christmas. Keeps in touch all the time." Residents also underscored the centrality of friendships formed among themselves by dining together: "Yeah, everybody sits at their own table of people and I like that. … Cause you may get somebody you're not the best friend of" (Interview with resident).

The pleasure of intergenerational activities

Opportunities for bringing older residents together with younger children on a regular basis were viewed as crucial for enhancing residents' well-being in all the homes we visited. Most often this occurred through regular family visits. The Volunteer Coordinator at one home observed:

'So, we have a number of younger kids and grandkids who come with their parent or grandparent. So, if they're under 13 they cannot register as a volunteer, they cannot volunteer on their own, but they can come in with their family. And so that happens quite often that the family members will come in and volunteer together. … The seniors like that because they love seeing some really young people around.'

The presence of children could transform a unit, a hired personal companion said: "It makes such a difference here, because, you know, when a family bring in young children all the people cling to them." A daughter whose mother lived in another home agreed. Bringing children and grandchildren into the home was hugely important, she argued, not just for her mother but for the other residents on her floor. Referring to one of them, she said: "When her daughter brings her baby in with her it's just like Christmas morning." This home also had a children's daycare on the premises which, according to the home's Recreational Director, made a huge difference: "We have a daycare right there … often. … We can wheel [the residents] over to see new babies." In this rural home, where most residents had family members living nearby, there were many opportunities for unplanned informal intergenerational contact. As one resident boasted, "I have one [grandchild] from [town] that comes all the time. … One minute you're sitting alone, two minutes, the next minute the door opens and then they call you".

In a third home, located in a more urban setting, a volunteer who is a retired music teacher played an innovative role in organising a large-scale programme for connecting residents, on a weekly basis, with children under the age of four.

Called 'Sing, Move, Play', her programme, she told us, was in essence meant "to combat loneliness for seniors. … Especially for seniors who don't have family this is really nice because it brings in young children and the parents". Over a six-week period, a group of 30 to 40 of the home's residents were brought together in a large auditorium, in a circle, with young, pre-school children and their parents to share activities together. The children were encouraged to present each resident with a gift which they could play with together, or a song which they could sing together. The volunteer described its powerful impact on one resident:

'I've got a picture of her actually because they've taken pictures sometimes of her holding a scarf and moving a scarf with the young children, and she's kind of brushing the scarf and she was as joyous as anything even though a few minutes ago she was in her room and she was miserable.'

In another example of a promising practice, a

'little toddler got up and sang in the centre and [a resident] said, "Oh that's the same song that I know of! Twinkle Twinkle Little Star", and he sang it all by himself. He said, "I wanna sing it!" and so he did a solo and everybody clapped at the end for him.' (Interview with volunteer)

'Sing, Move, Play' created many opportunities for fostering interdependence across generations, a 'win-win' experience for both the seniors and the children.

Getting residents out of their rooms

In all three facilities, volunteers, family members and residents played a critical role in helping residents get to activities and appointments both inside and outside the home. A special programme and volunteer manager in one NH stated that over the course of her career an increasingly small percentage of residents were able to participate in excursions outside the home:

> 'When I first started as a recreationist most of our residents were the kind of people that you would see living in retirement homes today. Most of them walked, some of them drove their own cars, a lot of them were fairly independent, so if there was an exercise class they would come to the exercise class. Now, I would say about 80 per cent of our residents require us to go and get them and take them to an activity, they require more support in the activities, they require sort of lower functioning activities, or activities where we provide assistance for them to be able to do things.'

This transformation in the ability of residents to go out on their own, or get to an activity with the help of staff, means that the unpaid work of volunteers is crucial: "Absolutely, we couldn't take the residents out if we didn't have volunteers go with us" (Interview with special programme and volunteer manager).

Volunteers in all three Ontario homes talked about how much they enjoyed taking residents who were able to do so, out shopping. "[M]aybe they don't have a family member but they want to shop," said one volunteer. Volunteers also helped residents stay in contact with outside government agencies. A senior staff member at one home provided some telling examples:

> 'So a volunteer came and picked up all the paperwork because it couldn't be mailed, it had to be delivered in person … it could only be delivered to City Hall. So this volunteer, we put her in a taxicab. I don't know what we would do without our volunteers. … So … unpaid work is really big here.' (Interview with resident care liaison manager)

In one home, a resident talked about introducing new residents to an outside Salvation Army workshop that specialised in pet therapy for seniors:

'Oh yes, I work in the Salvation Army on Tuesdays. They have like an old school and everybody goes in there, but our week was last week and we have a chance to take somebody that's never been there before and teach them what to do, and if they would like to bring somebody with them, they can bring them in and show them everything that they learnt to do and how we do it.'

An 80-year-old volunteer was praised for "help[ing] out in the barbershop taking people back and forth" (Interview with family council member). Volunteers took pride in "[taking] people back and forth to music, or I take them to bingo or choir or whatever, ice cream, you know. Those are things we can do as volunteers" (Interview with family council member). Family members played a similar role. "I'm in the choir, so I volunteer taking residents back and forth for music" (Interview with family member). As a daughter recalled:

'I could come after dinner or at dinner and then take him to an evening social event. And usually because I knew the people on the floor by that point I could help various people. Like, Dad was in a chair but if there was a couple of people in walkers we could go together up the halls.' (Interview with daughter and family council member)

A sister captured the simple pleasure of getting her brother outside: "I bring peanuts, he feeds the squirrels and he loves that." But she was uncertain whether she could do the same for other residents on her brother's unit. "Sometimes I wonder, though, if some of the other residents, like can you invite them to go for a walk?"

Some family members fought strenuously against their relatives being confined to secure units because they realised how much would be lost if they were cut off from the world outside the nursing home's walls:

'There's no activity here on most floors that I see except a half hour here and there. But the rest of the time they're in the activity room or the TV room just sitting there. Some of them [are] watching programmes that I'm sure that just go in one ear and out the other ... I like to take her out every day if I can. And there's a nice garden here. And ... they're pushing me to get [her] out of that [downstairs] floor ... because she lost the ability to walk. And I resisted and resisted, because I didn't want her to be parked.' (Interview with spouse)

Volunteers and family members were relied upon regularly to transport residents inside or outside their homes for social activities or for key events such as medical appointments, underscoring the reality of understaffing at all three facilities. As one spouse told us, "the staff didn't … have the time". Another family member stressed the importance of taking her relative to doctors' appointments herself because "it's far easier for me to talk to the doctor directly than to get a written report". A volunteer in the same home agreed that there were simply not enough staff available to help residents leave their rooms: "I think I would have a number of people who don't get out of their rooms and have the volunteers go and bring them down for coffee or tea because they don't come down because they're not – don't have anybody to bring them."

The shift from paid to unpaid work

The interviews in this chapter highlight five critical ways in which family members, volunteers, staff and residents themselves provided crucial unpaid work across a variety of boundaries to support the quality of social life in nursing homes. The interviews show that this unpaid work has been crucial to protecting and enhancing the quality of life of this increasingly frail population of residents by providing opportunities for meaningful social relationships and social activities. The interviews also underscore the urgent need for increased staffing and greater attention to the voices of family members, volunteers and residents themselves to ensure safer and more dignified lives for Ontario's expanding nursing home population. As Sandvoll et al (2020, pp 2 and 4) argue, 'activities contribute to [nursing home residents'] wellbeing and dignity' but nursing homes 'do not systematically document residents' individual needs for activities, and staff state they lack the time to support individual activities'. The result, as our Ontario findings demonstrate, is a shift in responsibility from paid care work towards a wide array of unpaid contributions from volunteers and family members in order to sustain the quality of resident lives, a conclusion which echoes and elaborates on current research from other jurisdictions (see, for instance, Skinner et al, 2018).

COVID-19 had caused almost 4,000 nursing home resident deaths in Ontario by the end of April 2021, accounting for 61 per cent of all COVID-19 deaths in the province – one of the highest percentages in the world. This shocking reality underscored the enormous vulnerabilities of residents living in long-term care in Ontario (Ontario, 2021, p 1). Prior to the pandemic, the significance of the unpaid work of family members and volunteers, overwhelmingly women, to making "the]difference between survival and living" (as the wife of a resident quoted earlier put it) for residents in care was already critical. When COVID-19 infection control protocols excluded them from entering care homes, the quality of life of the residents deteriorated catastrophically. This outcome not only emphasises the urgency of dramatic increases in the numbers and job security of paid staff. It also highlights the need for new collaborative strategies to expand the voices of family members, family councils and volunteers in the social life, daily activities and operation of Ontario's nursing homes, as called for by Family Councils Ontario (2022, pp 1–8).

References

Ågotnes, G. and Øye, C. (2018) Facilitating resident community in nursing homes: A slippery slope? An analysis on collectivistic and individualistic approaches, *Health*, 22(5): 469–82.

Ågotnes G., Moholt J.-M. and Blix, B.H. (2021) From volunteer work to informal care by stealth: A "new voluntarism" in social democratic health and welfare services for older adults, *Ageing and Society*: 1–17, https://doi.org/10.1017/S0144686X21001598

Barken, R., Daly, T. and Armstrong, P. (2016) Family matters: The work and skills of family/friend carers in long-term residential care, *Journal of Canadian Studies*: 50(2): 321–47.

Family Councils Ontario (2022) Guidance for Family Councils and Long-Term Care Home Collaboration, Final Report 30 April 2021, Available from: fco.ngo/resources/guidance-for-family-councils-and-long-term-care-home-collaboration

Ferreira, K. (2021) 'Ontario's Long-Term Care COVID-19 Commission releases its final report' [Blog] 23 June, Koskie Minsky LLP, Available from: https://kmlaw.ca/ontarios-long-term-care-covid-19-commission-releases-its-final-report/

Freedman, A. and Nicolle, J. (2020) Social isolation and loneliness: The new geriatric giants, *Canadian Family Physician*, 66(3): 176–82.

Grenade, L. and Boldy, D. (2008) Social isolation and loneliness among older people: Issues and future challenges in community and residential settings, *Australian Health Review*, 32(3): 468–78, doi:10.1071/ah080468

Grootegoed E., Van Barneveld, E. and Duyvendak, J.W. (2015) What is customary about customary care? How Dutch welfare policy defines what citizens have to consider "normal" care at home, *Critical Social Policy*, 35: 110–31.

Hande, M., Taylor, D. and Keefe, J. (2021) The role of volunteers in enhancing resident quality of life in long-term care: Analyzing policies that may enable or limit this role, *Canadian Journal on Aging / La Revue canadienne du vieillissement*: 1–12, doi:10.1017/S0714980821000106

Harmer, B. and Orrell, M. (2008) What is meaningful activity for people with dementia living in care homes? A comparison of the views of older people with dementia, staff, and family carers, *Aging and Mental Health*, 12(5): 548–58.

Knight, T. and Mellor, D. (2007) Social inclusion of older adults in care: Is it just a question of providing activities? *International Journal of Qualitative Studies on Health and Well-Being*, 2(2): 76–85.

Kröger, T. and Leinonen, A. (2012) Transformation by stealth: The retargeting of home care services in Finland, *Health and Social Care in the Community*, 20: 319–27.

Lowndes, R., Struthers, J. and Ågotnes, G. (2020) Social participation in long-term residential care: Case studies from Canada, Norway, and Germany, *Canadian Journal on Aging/La Revue canadienne du vieillissement*, 40(1): 1–18.

Ontario (2021) Ontario's Long-Term Care COVID-19 Commission, Final Report 30 April 2021, Available from: files.ontario.ca/mltc-ltcc-final-report-en-2021-04-30.pdf, pp 1–402.

Sandvoll, A.M, Hjertenes, A.M. and Board, M. (2020) Perspectives on activities in nursing homes, *International Practice Development Journal*, 10, 1–12, https://doi.org/10.19043/ipdj.10Suppl.006

Skinner, M., Sogstad, M. and Tingvold, L. (2018) Voluntary work in the Norwegian long-term care sector: Complementing or substituting formal services?, *European Journal of Social Work*, 22(6): 1–13.

Smith, J.M. (2012) Portraits of loneliness: Emerging themes among community-dwelling older adults, *Journal of Psychosocial Nursing and Mental Health Services*, 50(4): 34–9, doi:10.3928/02793695-20120306-04

Smith, N., Towers, A., Palmer, S., Beecham, J. and Welch, E. (2018) Being occupied: Supporting 'meaningful activity' in care homes for older people in England, *Ageing and Society*, 38(11): 2218–2240.

Suragarn, U., Hain, D. and Pfaff, G. (2021) Approaches to enhance social connection in older adults: An integrative review of literature, *Aging and Health Research*, 1(3): 1–9, https://doi.org/10.1016/j.ahr.2021.100029

Theurer, K., Mortenson, W., Stone, R., Suto, M., Timoren, V. and Rozanova, J. (2015) The need for a social revolution in residential care, *Journal of Aging Studies*, 35: 201–10.

Ulmanen, P. and Szebehely, M. (2015) From the state to the family or to the market? Consequences of reduced residential eldercare in Sweden, *International Journal of Social Welfare*, 24: 81–92.

Van Regenmortel, S., De Donder, L., Dury, S., Smetcoren, A.-S., De Witte, N. and Verté, D. (2016) Social exclusion in later life: A systematic review of the literature, *Population Ageing*, 9: 15–344, https://doi.org/10.1007/s12062-016-9145-3

5

Residents who care: rethinking complex care and disability relations in Ontario nursing homes

Janna Klostermann

FIELD DIARY

4 April 2018

In an activities room, I chatted with a resident, 'Ralph', who said, "I'd love to speak with you, but before we start, I have a problem with my hand. Perhaps you could help me out". He worked the joke, giving a lead up. He then held out a fake plastic hand on the end of his finger. It was a subversive joke – poking fun at task-based body care and at people continually asking how he's doing. The joke seemed to be a way to cope with his changing body and with the care apparatus he was part of, as he also noted that he does have arthritis, that his fingers are in pain.

I wrote the above field note following an encounter I had at an urban Ontario nursing home. Cracking jokes seemed to offer 'Ralph' a way to negotiate his circumstances in a context where residents are sometimes understood as 'bed-and-bodywork' (Gubrium, 1975), as 'routine work' (Paterniti, 2003) or as 'institutional bodies' that fit into institutional structures (Weirsma, 2010; Wiersma and Dupuis, 2010; see also Chapter 3). Ralph used his 'material', worked with what he had. His use of humour provides one illustration of how residents 'reconcil[e] tensions between care needs and concerns about burdening others' (Barken, 2017; see also Aronson, 2002) in sites where they increasingly rely on the unpaid care of others. With a prop in hand, and time to 'set up' the joke, Ralph creatively and strategically acknowledged and negotiated his own care needs. Humour was one way to play it. And in this chapter, I explore a range of other ways in which residents negotiate complex relations of support. I ask: How do residents navigate, negotiate and make sense of their own and others' care needs, and how are their practices socially and organisationally mediated?

This chapter engages with and aims to contribute to a robust tradition of care scholarship that attends to the everyday health work, life work or self-management work that people accessing care do (Mykhalovskiy and Smith, 1994; Aronson, 2002; Lombardo et al, 2014; Hurl and Klostermann, 2019). For instance, Lombardo et al (2014) noted women that needing home care put work into 'mobilising financial, social and interpersonal resources; living out shortfalls by making do, doing without, and emotional self-management; and avoiding illness and maintaining health' (p 575). Aronson's (2002) research on home care also shines a light on the work of those receiving services. In her study, one person noted that 'the government said: "Well you should get family"' (p 408), while another woman said her case manager had advised her to recruit a neighbour to help her with her evening eye drops (p 409). The onus was on them to figure out how to get their care needs met, with many indicating they did not want to be a burden. One woman receiving home care described a barely palatable meal: "But I ate it; I didn't want to hurt her feelings" (p 412).

Some researchers have found that care home residents work to 'make the best' of it (Kahn, 1999) or downplay their struggles to family and friends (Wilson, 1997). They learn to conform or become part of routines to survive, and to try not to come across as needy, difficult or troublesome (Wiersma, 2010, p 432). All of this takes time and energy, as they participate in, learn about and even resist everyday institutional routines. Nursing home residents today often enter care facilities with higher acuity levels and more complex care needs. Further, residents have varying care needs, health and mental health diagnoses (Giosa et al, 2014), and require different levels of support in performing activities of daily living (Patterson, 2016), which shapes the relationships residents have with one another, and gives rise to tensions that need to be unpacked and handled.

Offering a lens for exploring negotiated and coordinated dimensions of care, Armstrong (2019) defines the 'right (not) to care' as the right to provide or not provide some forms of care work, to receive or not receive care, with conditions that make those rights and forms of work possible and even rewarding (see also Armstrong and Klostermann, in press). Such an understanding of the 'right (not) to care' is informed both by the work of care ethicists, who take seriously the notion that 'everyone is entitled to receive adequate care throughout life' (Tronto, 2006, p 19; see also Daly, 2013), and by feminist political economists, who are attentive to how women are conscripted or coerced into caring, with 'diverse forms of coercion that have induced women to assume responsibility for caring for family members and that have tracked poor, racial minority and immigrant women into positions entailing caring for others' (Glenn, 2010, p 5). The 'right (not) to care' is a matter of gender and intersectional inequities, with gender, racial, class/income and citizenship relations shaping who can access care, who is tracked into care roles and who is prevented from being able to care (for example, without adequate support or resources). In terms of choice, it's notable that unpaid care is often a result of coercion and isn't always something people have a choice in whether to provide or not, particularly when the welfare state is not able to meet people's needs (Overgaard, 2019; Armstrong and Klostermann, in press).

This chapter explicates organisational relations in several Ontario nursing homes, and circulating narratives of care and disability, through an analysis of how residents make sense of, respond to and negotiate their own and others' care needs. I focus on the contributions residents make to care as they foster and navigate relationships and negotiate complex relations of support in the context of privatisation and late neoliberalism. I bring into view care and social glue activities that residents engage in and create, looking at the work that residents do to strategically respond to their own and others' care needs. My analysis captures the dynamics of paid and unpaid care work in Ontario nursing homes, while also shining a light on *negotiated* practices, meanings and relations of care and disability. Following Smith (2005), I apply an expanded definition of 'work' to account for 'anything done by people that takes time and effort, that they mean to do, that is done under definite conditions' (pp 151–2). I attend in particular to social glue activities 'that sustain individuals and communities and the bonds between them' (Baines et al, 2020; see also Fraser, 2016, p 2). I also recognise that such activities 'contain an eliminable personal element. They are, by definition, interpersonal, involving intersubjective communication and in some cases, physical touching' (Fraser, 2016, p 7; see also Baines et al, 2020, p 455). With a focus on how residents negotiate the circumstances of their lives, including in everyday talk, my aim is to link their practices to social and organisational relations, while also elaborating on how those relations are and can be reshaped (Klostermann, 2019, 2021).

I draw on rapid, team-based, site-switching ethnographic research (Armstrong and Lowndes, 2018) conducted at three non-profit, municipal and unionised care facilities in central and eastern Ontario. In keeping with other chapters in this collection, I use feminist political economy to attend to, theorise and explicate the unpaid work that people do in care homes as a form of privatisation that can be attributed to inadequate public sector support for care (Armstrong and Armstrong, 2019). I also use some rhetorical analysis tools to analyse how people framed their work or positioned themselves in our conversations, which helps me to reveal dimensions of social organisation in everyday talk (Klostermann, 2019). I shine a light on organisational logics and relations of care, aging and disability. In Ontario, it's not just that an aging population has increased demand for care, but that a lack of investment and a shortage of beds has kept people on waiting lists, which means they are entering later in life with more complex needs. With privatisation and neoliberal self-governance (Petersen and Lupton, 1996), the onus falls on individuals to remain healthy, practise self-care or take responsibility for their own and others' care needs. At care homes stretched thin, *individuals* are left providing unpaid or additional work to pick up the slack.

Care work, social bonds and the resident who said "no": situating residents' embodied practices and possibilities

In what follows, I identify contradictions and complexities in residents' contributions, considering how residents variously negotiate, coordinate or provide care for themselves and others. Along the way, following research that considers institutional practices that shape how care workers relate to residents (Weirsma and Dupuis, 2010), I elaborate how residents' practices are organisationally mediated, with staff playing an important role in overseeing, facilitating and at times limiting residents' contributions and social connections.

> FIELD DIARY
>
> *4 April 2018*
>
> The woman in the wheelchair was making rounds around the hallway, with her head down and moving the chair with her feet. She came back to our circle and was confused: she didn't know where someone was and she was worried about him. The ladies [two residents] were quick to reassure her they didn't know who she was talking about but they were sure he was fine.

Written by a researcher on our team, the fieldnote above captures one of many examples of a resident asking for support, and of other residents stepping in to notice and respond to that person's needs. 'Residents care for each other in meaningful ways that make them feel good' is how the researcher quoted earlier put it. As we documented in our research, some residents mentioned finding meaning in supporting others, yet others talked about struggling to set limits on the care they provided. As Glenn (2010) writes, care work can involve a range of ordinary work related to providing direct (physical and emotional) support for a person, maintaining physical surroundings (such as by cleaning up) and fostering relationships and networks. Like care workers in a study by Baines et al (2020), residents recreate 'social bonds ... in various forms and iterations' and 'reweave[e] the social fabric through care and relationship' despite austerity and other life challenges. They engage in care activities and in activities to sustain relationships.

The following is an interaction I participated in and wrote about that speaks to how residents, as they actively notice and respond to others' needs, contribute to the social fabric of long-term care:

'I was mingling in the dining room with two residents, Lou and Helen, and one of the residents' daughters, Karen. Karen joked that Lou was the "den mother" and kept tabs on her mom, Helen. She also mentioned how hard it was to see that her mom wasn't talking today, as she was usually chatty. The three of us chatted away, while Helen kept quiet. "Helen, are you from the area?" I said, peeling myself out of the conversation with the others and purposely making eye contact with her. We all just waited, just dangled there. No one spoke for Helen, but Karen eventually said, ★slowly★, "Mom? She's asking if you are from the area?" For the first time in our conversation, Helen turned to look at me, smiling and holding my gaze, but she still didn't speak. As we waited, her friend Lou said, "She's from Ottawa. Helen's always dressed to the hilts. You should see her paintings; she's an artist. Her paintings are out of this world". It was less about what she said, and more that she said it. I understood Lou's response to be a way to care for Helen and for Helen's daughter, Karen. She put it on the record that Helen meant something to her. Lou also went on to say how much she'd enjoyed connecting with both Helen and Karen. Lou talked about how Karen brought in the good grapes. Karen noted that she had also brought in a box of wine for movie night. Helen smiled along. Lou mentioned that Helen's daughter, Karen, had hosted her for a holiday dinner, before Karen joked warmly, "Well, I kept asking and eventually she caved".'

There was a sense of ease, vitality and even joy, as they riffed and responded to one another. This was just one example of a resident extending care to another resident and her family member. It was also an example that illustrates how relationships are not static; they change over time, including with regards to residents' health, family circumstances and social context (Keefe and Fancey, 2000). While some examples were easy to write about, reading them alongside other stories residents told (reproduced below) reveals complexities and contradictions in residents' care work and social glue activities.

"Oh yes, if they need help, I'll – I'll do it," Bev, a resident in her eighties, said. She took a lot of care to position herself as a caring person. When asked for an example of how she supported other residents, she said, "Oh, like they can't seem to walk too far, so you take their arm and sit them down". While Bev presented herself as someone who would willingly and gladly offer to help others, she also mentioned she had had to set limits on the support she could provide to a particular resident. As she said, "But that's not my job and I've told her," she seemed to distinguish between supporting someone voluntarily and on her own terms, and having it seen as her "job". While she didn't elaborate, her story had me wondering how much would have led up to that – how many moments of volunteering or being willing to help had led up to her setting limits and saying no, "that's not my job". A point made by Weirsma and Dupuis (2010, p 285) – that residents often learn that they are 'not the only ones with care needs' – would perhaps seem like an understatement from Bev's perspective, as it wasn't just that she was struggling to get her own needs met, but that she was also tasked with negotiating the needs of others. Her account also speaks to the changing boundaries between tasks that seem meaningful or nourishing and those that seem burdensome or oppressive.

The support that Bev and other residents provide (or decide whether to provide or not) is organisationally mediated. Low staffing levels leave gaps in care, with resident care needs which can then either be left unmet or filled by unpaid work. When filled by the unpaid care work of other residents who are living in the facility and seemingly always on hand, those same needs can then result in tensions or in dilemmas residents have to negotiate around whether or when to set limits or say no. Depending on how paid work is organised, managed and staffed, unpaid work might become necessary, which gives rise at times to deeply felt interpersonal negotiations. If there had been more paid staff on the floor, perhaps Bev wouldn't have been put in a situation where she'd face as many requests or would have to set limits.

In fact, Bev herself elaborated on how paid staff can make a difference in limiting the care that residents are asked to provide. When asked whether she helped anybody in the dining room, Bev said, "Well, see, we have enough staff that they're taking care of ones that can't feed themselves, right? I'd help them if they wanted me. Sometimes you're told mind your own business". Bev's point was an important one, as it highlights how the mandated hours of care per day for residents and the number of staff on a shift shape residents' 'care negotiation' practices, as well as the nature of relationships between residents. It was also notable that even though she had once worked in housekeeping, she wasn't being approached to help with that work. "No, I'm out of that," Bev said, laughing. What was also striking to me was that, even as she lived in a place where she herself was eligible for 24/7 care, she too upheld and negotiated gendered imperatives to care with the statement "I'd help them if they wanted me". Circulating narratives of 'care' that link caring about someone with providing direct care for someone were apparent in her account. Women residents who talked about how their lives had been defined by caring for others or by volunteering were tasked with figuring out how to live or whether to hold back.

A younger resident, Wally, also told stories that helped to illustrate how the care and social glue activities he engaged in were socially organised. Supporting others was a source of pride for Wally, who had moved into the care home after living in a psychiatric facility for a couple of decades. He introduced himself to researchers on our team as a community builder and mentioned that he had been "blessed with a really good life" and that he wanted to be "able to make a contribution to other people". As I spoke to him while he was pedalling on an exercise bike, he also put a value on staying healthy, noting that he was trying to improve his physical fitness and memory. "I try and rewatch *Jeopardy* to improve my mind," he said. When asked what changes he'd like to see in the care home where he lived, he noted that he would like to have "all the staff wear their name tags out not in" so that he could "try to remember everybody's name", He said, "It's not so much my insecurity that I don't know their names; it's the fact that I just wanna respect them". He expressed how important it was for him to connect with and invest in others. "Sometimes it's as simple as saying 'Hi'," Wally explained. In speaking of trying to help staff, he said, "When I can, I try to take dishes over and garbage and things like that and give it to them to deal with". When Wally was asked whether staff were happy when he took dishes over, whether they appreciated the help, he said, "Yeah. Oh yeah, well, I did it once and it was OK. I did it twice, and I nearly dropped it. *Enough of that!* [laughs] Don't let me drop dishes, that's for sure". While it was unclear whether by "Enough of that", he meant that he was asked to stop carrying his dishes up, our interviews with staff confirmed that they often needed to oversee or set limits on residents "helping out".

Staff play a role in facilitating, overseeing and limiting residents' contributions (see Chapter 2). 'Allie', a recreation therapist, mentioned that she put thought into helping residents contribute to the running of recreational programmes and life in the care home. Speaking of an exercise class, she said, "There's one lady who gets up and helps me pass out the weights". She also mentioned others who helped to set up and clean up for events. She said, "When we have opportunity for set up for like parties and stuff, we'll bring some people out to help set the tables". Part of what Allie elaborated on was how much work was involved on her part to discern who could contribute and in what ways. Allie said, "When I bring a new person into programming, I try and sit them near someone who would be interested in talking to them, and introduce them". Sandra, another recreational therapist, explained, "[Y]ou know who to sit a newer person with for sure!" They took care to observe residents and to oversee residents' care and social glue practices, which could only happen over time as staff got to know others. All of this illustrates the importance of continuity, as getting to know the residents and supporting them takes time.

Staff also talked about monitoring and setting limits on residents' contributions, such as when they had concerns about health, safety and general well-being or when they observed tensions between some residents. Such a finding is supported by research that found staff focused on issues of safety and risk (Weirsma, 2010). In her work as a recreational therapist, Allie stated she tried "not to let [residents] touch the baking too much" as she was "concerned about health and hygiene". She mentioned that she monitored residents' contributions to ensure there was "consent" and a "conversation" such as with residents pushing others around in wheelchairs. As she said, "If the resident's not looking distressed that's being pushed around, then it's fine, but, you know, sometimes you have to get involved. [I'll be] like, 'Oh no, no, leave her alone, she's happy where she is'". Allie also referenced past conflicts that had led her to limit some residents' participation in certain tasks. For instance, she stopped inviting a woman resident to help set up "who used to be very much in charge of everything" and would "boss around" volunteers and staff, "telling [them] how to do it and that [they're] doing it wrong". As Allie said, "[L]ike the tables were in the wrong spot, the chairs were in the wrong spot, this is not how you set the table". She told another story about a resident who came to "help them decorate" but then stole their "decorations and [kept] them in his room". "And I said, 'No, go away. You can't come in here'". So, while staff often expressed ideals about having "residents at the front" (as one director of nursing put it), they weren't afraid to hold particular/individual residents accountable or to limit some contributions to support collective interests. This too took work and shows how paid work impacts on residents' practices and relationships.

At times it sounded as though staff were humouring residents (such as when Allie noted that some residents "think they're helping, [but] they're not really helping" or when a director of nursing talked about a resident who organised the desks of staff members, and mentioned that it "was even funnier" when the resident later came back to check to see if her desk was still organised). Yet, part of what staff put on the record was that they encouraged residents' participation in care, as "it gives them something to do and something meaningful" (as Allie put it). More than "letting" residents care just for fun, this work was often about providing a sense of meaning and community. Further, Allie did give examples of help from residents that was very much welcome and did seem to lighten the load of paid workers such as in speaking of residents escorting or "portering" others down the halls or of a resident who would get started on doing dishes while Allie was baking. As she said, one woman "starts washing the dishes and I don't even have to wash the dishes after".

Further calling attention to social relations and meanings of disability and care, staff and residents also elaborated on how residents' complex needs shaped their own and others' practices, relationships and understandings. In speaking of residents who were easier to sit with, Sandra, another recreational therapist, mentioned that most residents weren't in a position to "take [others] under [their] wing" or "show [them] around". As she said, "there's so many people who don't have that capability as much any more. … There's some people who certainly could. … But not as many as I'd like". This was often something residents also called attention to. Doreen, a resident in her nineties, indicated that she got along well with others, before noting, "Mind you, I don't bother with a lot of them because they've got Alzheimer's and dementia and so on". While she added that she had "hundreds of friends" outside of the facility", she said, "I don't have a lot of friends in here because you can't have, there's so much Alzheimer's and dementia and so on". Doreen's point about how residents' care needs and mental health and health diagnoses shape the quality or nature of relationships speaks to the changing resident populations noted earlier (Giosa et al, 2014). There are clear links to social policies or inadequate public sector support for care that see residents entering care later in life and with higher care needs.

It's also worth thinking about how Doreen and other residents have limited access to critical discourses or strategies that would offer alternative ways of making sense of and orienting to disability. A clear example of that was in the account of a woman resident, Betty, who said:

> 'Um, now mind you, uh, this, sounds like I'm a little bit conceited, I don't mean it conceited at all, I'm just telling you the truth. I am one of their better patients because I'm in good health, I'm in real good health, I don't have an ache or a pain anywhere in my body. And I'm 92 years of age.'

With an "um" and an "uh", and with her worries about sounding conceited, I was struck by her lack of access to critical discourses or circulating narratives that would invite more expansive ways of living with and orienting to disability or "bad" health, for example by regarding them as sites of joy, meaning-making, relationality or critical and creative potential. As Chivers' (2013, 2021) work underscores, circulating narratives of care, aging and disability are significant and affect late life relationships.

Taken together, residents' practices (such as to ask for care, care for themselves and others or make sense of their own or others' care needs) are shaped through inadequate public sector services and through circulating narratives of care, aging and disability. While the issues of staff shortages or of working short are clear from workers' accounts of bigger workloads and more residents to support with more complex needs, and are clear in that family carers are often called on to provide more care, they are also evident in examples of residents making sense of and negotiating complexities of congregate care. Their stories highlight the importance of residents having choices in the care they receive, and the care they provide, which is about having adequate publicly provided paid care. Ensuring care is maintained as a collective responsibility and provided by the state (as is the case in Norway and Sweden) would take the pressure off residents and lessen tensions. Relatedly, there is a need for alternative storylines, scripts or circulating narratives to help people with orienting to care and disability, and with navigating, negotiating and expressing the complexities of their everyday lives.

Concluding remarks

Drawing on ethnographic research conducted in three Ontario-based nursing homes, this chapter reflected on the 'right (not) to care' through a sociological analysis of residents' practices and relationships, as they are socially and organisationally mediated. My focus was on how residents foster relationships and negotiate their own and others' care needs, including by doing unpaid care work for others, in the context of privatisation and late neoliberalism. We traced residents' practices, making links to how staff and others play a role in facilitating and limiting residents' contributions. Low funding and low staffing levels leave gaps in care, care work undone and care needs 'unmet' or needing to be filled by unpaid labour. These conditions, along with circulating narratives about care needs or disability, set the stage for residents' unpaid care, social glue and boundary-setting practices, as well as their critical insights and jokes. As we've explored, practices, relations and meanings of 'care' change over time and are actively negotiated. That which is meaningful, joyful or consensual can morph into something burdensome, oppressive and constraining.

The boundaries between paid and unpaid work are boundaries that nursing home residents actively negotiate. The onus is on individual residents to creatively get their care needs met such as by seeking out the support of other residents or stepping in to provide care to others. 'Unmet' care needs can give rise to tensions that need to be recognised and handled. Not only do staff and family carers 'pick up the slack' at homes stretched thin, residents also put time, energy and effort into navigating these relations. This unpaid work not only takes time on their part, but also involves coordinated work from paid and unpaid carers, who need the time and conditions to be able to notice, respond to and support residents in engaging in meaningful ways. With their on-the-ground experiences and knowledge of care, and their creative and critical potential, residents negotiate meanings and relations of care and disability, finding ways to respond to their own and others' care needs, and to build or rethink relationships.

References

Armstrong, P. (2019) 'The feminization of the care labor force?', Paper presented at Global Carework Summit, 10 June University of Toronto.

Armstrong, P., Amaratunga, C., Bernier, J., Grant, K., Pederson, A. and Willson, K. (eds) (2002) *Exposing Privatization: Women and Health Care Reform*, Garamond Press.

Armstrong, P. and Armstrong, H. (eds) (2019) *The Privatization of Care: The Case of Nursing Homes*, Routledge.

Armstrong, P. and Lowndes, R. (eds) (2018) *Creative Teamwork: Developing Rapid, Site-switching Ethnography*, Oxford University Press.

Armstrong, P. and Klostermann, J. (in press) Unpaid work in public places: Nursing homes in times of Covid-19, in M. Duffy, A. Armenia and K. Price-Glynn (eds) *Confronting the Global Care Crisis During COVID-19: Past Problems, New Issues, and Pathways to Change*, Rutgers.

Aronson, J. (2002) Elderly people's accounts of home care rationing: Missing voices in long-term care policy debates, *Ageing & Society*, 22(4): 399–418.

Baines, D., Cunningham, I., Kgaphola, I. and Mthembu, S. (2020) Nonprofit care work as social glue: Creating and sustaining social reproduction in the context of austerity/late neoliberalism, *Affilia*, 35(4): 449–65.

Barken, R. (2017) Reconciling tensions: needing formal and family/friend care but feeling like a burden, *Canadian Journal on Aging / La Revue canadienne du vieillissement*, 36(1): 81–96.

Chivers, S. (2013) Care, culture and creativity: A disability perspective on long-term residential care, in P. Armstrong and S. Braedley (eds) *Troubling Care: Critical Perspectives on Research and Practices*, Canadian Scholars' Press, pp 47–58.

Chivers, S. (2021) Old friends: Reimagining care relations through Helen Garner's *The Spare Room*, in *Contemporary Narratives of Ageing, Illness, Care*, Routledge, pp 163–76.

Daly, T. (2013) Imagining an ethos of care within policies, practices, and philosophy in P. Armstrong and S. Braedley (eds) *Troubling Care: Critical Perspectives on Research and Practices*, pp 33–45.

Doucet, A. and Klostermann, J. (in press) What and how are we measuring when we research gendered divisions of household work and care? Remaking the household portrait method into a care/work portrait, *Sociological Research Online*.

Fraser, N. (2016) Capitalism's crisis of care, *Dissent*, 63(4): 30–7.

Giosa, J.L., Stolee, P., Dupuis, S.L., Mock, S.E. and Santi, S.M. (2014) An examination of family caregiver experiences during care transitions of older adults, *Canadian Journal on Aging/La Revue canadienne du vieillissement*, 33(2): 137–153.

Glenn, E.N. (2010) *Forced to Care: Coercion and Caregiving in America*, Harvard University Press.

Gubrium, J.F. (1975) *Living and Dying at Murray Manor*, St. Martin's Press.

Hurl, C. and Klostermann, J. (2019) Remembering George W. Smith's 'life work': From politico-administrative regimes to living otherwise, *Studies in Social Justice*, 13(2): 262–82.

Kahn, D.L. (1999) Making the best of it: Adapting to the ambivalence of a nursing home environment, *Qualitative Health Research*, 9(1): 119–32.

Keefe, J., Fancey, P. (2000) The care continues: Responsibility for elderly relatives before and after admission to a long term care facility, *Family Relations*, 49(3): 235–44.

Klostermann, J. (2019) Altering imaginaries and demanding treatment: Women's AIDS activism in Toronto, 1980s–1990s, in J. White-Farnham, B. Finer and C. Molloy (eds) *Women's Health Advocacy: Rhetorical Ingenuity for the 21st Century*, Routledge, pp 177–90.

Klostermann, J. (2021) 'Care has limits: Women's moral lives and revised meanings of care work', Unpublished doctoral dissertation, Carleton University.

Lombardo, A., Angus, J., Lowndes, R., Cechetto, N., Khattak, S., Ahmad, F. and Bierman, A. (2014) Women's strategies to achieve access to health care in Ontario, Canada: A meta-synthesis, *Health and Social Care in the Community*, 22(6): 575–87.

Mykhalovskiy, E. and Smith, G.W. (1994) *Hooking Up to Social Services: A Report on the Barriers People Living with HIV/AIDS Face Assessing Social Services*, Community AIDS Treatment Information Exchange.

Overgaard, C. (2019) Rethinking volunteering as a form of unpaid work, *Nonprofit and Voluntary Sector Quarterly*, 48(1): 128–45.

Paterniti, D.A. (2003) Claiming identity in a nursing home, in J.F. Gubrium and J.A. Holstein (eds) *Ways of Aging*, Blackwell Publishing, pp 58–74.

Patterson, E. (2016) 'Examining variation in access to long-term home care services for Ontario Service', Unpublished doctoral dissertation, University of Toronto.

Petersen A. and Lupton D. (1996) *The New Public Health: Health and Self in the Age of Risk*, Sage.

Smith, D.E. (2005) *Institutional Ethnography: A Sociology for People*, Rowman Altamira.

Tronto, J. (2006) Vicious circles of privatized caring, in M. Hamington and D.C. Miller (eds) *Socializing Care: Feminist Ethics and Public Issues,* Rowman and Littlefield Publishers Inc, pp 3–26.

Wiersma, E.C. (2010) Life around ... : Staff's perceptions of residents' adjustment into long-term care, *Canadian Journal on Aging / La Revue canadienne du vieillissement*, 29(3): 425–34.

Wiersma, E. and Dupuis, S.L. (2010) Becoming institutional bodies: Socialization into a long-term care home, *Journal of Aging Studies*, 24(4): 278–91.

Wilson, S.A. (1997) The transition to nursing home life: A comparison of planned and unplanned admissions, *Journal of Advanced Nursing*, 26: 864–71

6

Family workers: the work and working conditions of families in nursing homes

Christine Streeter

Some people assume that nursing home care eliminates the need for family care, but our research in Ontario, Canada, shows otherwise.[1] This chapter examines the over-reliance on the unpaid work of families in Ontario nursing homes, with a focus on work processes, working conditions and worker protections and supports (or their absence). Through a document scan analysis and a focus on the labour of family/friends (Baumbusch and Phinney, 2013), I move from identifying the range of work families do, to looking at how families are understood in organisational policies, procedures and processes, to discussing how conditions of work intersect with conditions of care. Along the way, I develop the concept of 'family worker', which offers a lens to account for family contributions in nursing homes. In conjunction with adequate staffing, I suggest this politicised concept be used in practice to facilitate staff collaboration with family workers in order to have the work of the latter recognised and their conditions of work improved. Such collaboration would include the development of work processes, means of documenting the work and resources to improve conditions of work and support relations between staff and families.

A range of scholarship attends to the work, skill and knowledge of families who support their relatives in nursing homes (Chapters 2 and 4). Following the move to a nursing home, available family/friends do significant unpaid care work to support residents and to contribute to care provision (Gladstone et al, 2006). This work is skilled care work, including much more than interpersonal care, and it deserves recognition and support (England et al, 2002; Armstrong, 2013). As Barken et al (2016) point out, there are discrepancies between how nursing home handbooks articulate family participation and what is done in practice. This chapter extends this research by orienting to families as workers (albeit unpaid), and by examining their working conditions. This is a timely area of investigation, with pandemic challenges and labour shortages underscoring the need for the dignified and coordinated post-pandemic care that families provide.

My central contribution is orienting to family/friends as family workers considering the implications of taking family workers' labour as work that deserves some protections, and supporting conditions to make it happen. I begin by tracing the range of work families do and analysing nursing home organisational documents, showing that they do not specify processes for family involvement with staff, residents and others or safety conditions for families. I then focus on the dynamics and interactions of family and staff work, suggesting that nursing homes move beyond the term 'communication' in describing family work processes to documenting these processes and developing structural conditions that ensure quality work and care for everyone involved.

Guided by feminist political economy (FPE), our team used ethnographic methods (Armstrong and Lowndes, 2018) to investigate whether and how family workers participated in care provision, how this care was considered, and with what effects for residents, paid staff and unpaid workers. FPE directs attention to the intersecting political, economic and social relations that both shape and undo hierarchies of privilege and oppression, including relations of race, class and gender (Luxton, 2006). With a historical materialist perspective, the approach makes human welfare central to the analysis, acknowledging that conditions of everyday life and the labour processes involved vary.

FPE aids this chapter to continue redefining the notion of work, understanding that unpaid labour is key to care. We assume unpaid work is work that deserves good working conditions. While paid workers have written agreements about safety conditions, unpaid family workers doing similar work in the same environment have none or very few, leaving the boundaries between paid and unpaid work both flexible and unprotected. Drawing on FPE concepts of unpaid and paid forms of work, this chapter seeks to make visible the unpaid skilled work done mainly by women (Armstrong, 2013). Attention to structures and relations in unpaid work done by families helps us to think through what working conditions, such as training, equipment, and health and safety might be needed for family workers in nursing homes. This skilled unpaid care work is deserving of respect and good conditions.

This chapter draws on organisational documents, interviews and fieldnotes from three Ontario, nursing homes: one urban site and two rural ones. At each site, the team gathered collective agreements, facility handbooks, guidelines, forms and policies that described processes and requirements for everyone involved in the home. A document scan analysis was completed (Bowen, 2009) by coding, highlighting and analysing 20 documents[2] relevant to the research question, 'How are family workers discussed or mentioned in organisation policies, procedures and processes in nursing homes?' (O'Leary, 2014). I also draw on an analysis of 20 interviews with family/friends and staff. All of this developed in conversation with the research team, which helped to shape the analysis and to ensure reflexive and rigorous research (Armstrong and Lowndes, 2018).

The multiple forms of family workers' unpaid work

Family workers make significant contributions to care provision in nursing homes (Gaugler, 2005). In Ontario nursing homes, low funding and low staffing levels mean that there are significant gaps in care left to be filled by unpaid labour, often through family involvement. These workers provide essential and supplementary care support, which is often 'encouraged and assumed' (Barken et al, 2016). Family workers, who are mostly women, respond to the needs of both residents and the nursing home. We found, through interviews and fieldwork, that the unpaid work Ontario families did in nursing homes occurred on three main levels: personalising care, coordinating care and advocating for care.

Personalising care

Personalising care involves the needs associated with clothing, laundry, food and housekeeping. The importance of these needs and the work involved are often invisible and undervalued (Koren, 2010; Armstrong and Day, 2020). Several family workers explained how they supported relatives by taking home and washing items of clothing or other items that required gentle laundering. This type of personalised care often takes time to coordinate with staff; for instance, to keep things labelled and organised to ensure these items don't get placed in the communal wash. Family workers also shared how they completed domestic tasks and personalized care when helping other residents. This type of work included social and community care. They described how they actively engaged with residents, often reporting how much they enjoyed this meaningful time. A director of care talked about a family member who worked in the dining room every morning: "We have a lady upstairs who, she's here every … she's getting everyone their coffee and their drinks. … She's part of the dining room and honestly, who would we get to sub in to do that?"

We witnessed the assumed involvement of family workers after the move to care, which places pressure on family workers to personalise tasks in nursing homes. One way family workers personalised care was by purchasing additional food and drink that brought joy to the residents and provided a sense of their individual self. One woman described bringing her mom "hot chocolate" and "some extra old cheese and some crackers 'cause that's what she likes". She also noted that the "budget doesn't allow them to have extra stuff like that here".

Coordinating care

Family workers also discussed spending their time coordinating additional forms of care that residents didn't receive in the nursing home. For instance, one director of care noted that staff oversaw what food families brought into the home. They said that with "communal living" and people "going in and out of rooms", the work involved ensuring staff "keep these items in the nursing station". Coordination is needed between family workers and staff if food is to be brought to the nursing station and used when a resident requires it. Another family member talked about "getting an emergency care doctor to come in and look after" her mom. The staff, she said, don't have the time: "They really don't. They care deeply about each person but the bells are ringing on the wall and people are just needing them all the time." Sometimes this additional care costs extra and families must pay for a private room or for foot care and medical care that is usually provided by the home. One family explained that they needed to bring in a care specialist, to attend to specific care needs, because the workers did not have time to attend to their mom.

In another interview, a family worker noted that her contributions to the nursing home included cleaning. This took her away from spending relational time with relatives and caused extra stress and worries: "If we could just get the bed issue settled, I will clean the floors, I will clean the mat, I will clean the toilet when it's dirty. Which happens fairly often. But if they would just do the bed – it has become, I suppose, the bugaboo for me, right?" Diminishing the stress caused by such problems (in this case the need for daily cleaning) would require a safe environment for family workers to discuss the issue with staff, and the ability for the nursing home to ensure they could solve the problem themselves.

Advocating for change

Family workers often advocate for and step in to support residents. A woman recalled how her husband moved in during a long weekend in September. She said she spent the weekend "bumbling around by myself, trying to find out how this whole business [worked]". She said, "It was all very new and confusing, and frustrating. So, we did not get off to, you know, the ideal start". Her advocacy work to push for new intake processes was motivated by her own experience. She now serves on the Admissions Committee and as a transitions volunteer, accompanying residents and families on the day of their arrival. She oversees the intake of residents into nursing home facilities. She recalled "working ... with the Admissions Office" to "streamline" the process, for example by giving families a checklist on the day of admission. These family workers also often act as an interface, communicating what new family workers, paid staff and new residents need to do and know. They help ensure ongoing care is provided, learning systems and monitoring and coordinating additional care, as well as advocating for other needs.

A family council is defined as 'an organized, self-led, self-determining, democratic group composed of family and friends of the residents of a nursing home' (Family Councils ON, nd), and we witnessed much unpaid labour by members of such groups. Although 'every home must have a Residents' Council', they are only required to have a family council 'if even one family member or person of importance (a friend or significant other) requests it' (Change Foundation, 2016, p 6). Like the Change Foundation (2016, p 12), we found family councils performed three main functions: enhancing the quality of life for residents, enhancing the quality of care for residents, and sharing information.

On paper: narrow depiction of working conditions

How are family workers mentioned in organisation policies, procedures and processes in nursing homes? From this document analysis, I found that nursing home organisational documents did not specify suitable processes for staff involvement with family workers. There was little description of working conditions, such as what family workers needed to do to relay important information to staff, or what type of equipment, or health or safety protections were available to families, and what they could and could not do with residents. Moreover, the encounter between the family worker and paid staff was rarely articulated in terms of labour processes, reflecting the assumption that family workers' unpaid work was voluntary rather than required.

How are families discussed?

When families were mentioned, there was a focus on (1) communication; (2) particular procedures (such as transitions into the home); and (3) a 'resident and family centred care approach' (which wasn't elaborated on). First, 'communication' was a key word. Organisational documents and policies encouraged communication between staff and residents' families, and 'establishing a good relationship' was highlighted. But there was no explanation of *how* this communication was to take place. Of course, communication is key within the nursing home setting; however, communication doesn't always equate to 'a good relationship', 'positive involvement' or a 'friendly and open atmosphere'. Further, the details or implementation of this communication such as who, how often, when and where were missing. The policy-oriented documents at these nursing homes emphasised the need to communicate with families 'effectively' and 'in a professional manner', while maintaining 'routine contact', 'responding appropriately in a timely manner' and 'utilizing family members as a key resource'.

Second, there was some mention of organisational procedures involving families. Employee and resident handbooks mentioned families when writing about institutional processes, such as transitions into care homes. For instance, one resident care handbook included details of policies that friends and family should know on everything from furniture and clothing to advocacy, so that family/friends could become familiar with them. In our research, a resident's sister shared details about her visits during the first two weeks of the transition from home to care. She explained that she visited her brother every day for several hours to ensure the transition went smoothly and that he was getting comfortable with the routine. These documents were critical to her understanding the home's policies and procedures, including when residents should go to the dining room for meals, how they should go for walks outside and how their rooms should be set up.

Third, a phrase used in two of the three homes' documents was a 'resident and family-centred care approach'. The documents didn't describe this approach, but rather explained that the homes and staff were to use this approach. Although residents and families were supposed to be at the centre of care, these documents did not detail exactly how this should take place, thereby failing to acknowledge the work of families.

What is missing?

From policies and reports to resident and employee handbooks, the ways that family workers are discussed in organisational texts do not reflect their contributions. In fact, there was little or no mention of families in strategic plans, priorities and quality improvement plans. When they were mentioned, such as in job descriptions, the documentation referred to staff communicating with families, without any discussion of the collaborative dimensions of their interactions and the ongoing involvement of family/ friends. Some texts talked abstractly about procedures or about resident and family care, but there was little specification of families' working conditions, rights and protections in the support they would need to carry out certain tasks.

Most organisational material does not acknowledge the contributions of families. A clear example was in employee job descriptions. In all three homes, the only job description that mentioned families was for the one for Registered Practical Nurse (RPN). Two of the homes provided a limited reference to involvement with families in recreational workers' job descriptions. Yet from our time in these homes, we found family workers to be in discussion with workers at all of the different levels at the home.

The smallest amount of discussion of families was in the documents that included future planning, such as annual reports, priorities in action and in quality improvement and quality improvement plans. Quality improvement plans did not discuss improvements related to families. But interestingly, when discussing how the nursing home could improve quality indicators, family involvement was frequently added to the list. For example, an objective to reduce pain for residents included an indicator measuring the percentage of residents whose pain worsened. The process for improving this indicator included redesigning a care plan for residents experiencing pain by involving family workers in the design of this plan. This illustrates how families are often drawn on, or relied upon, to attend to issues within the home. Additionally, some homes provided examples of the involvement of family workers in quality improvement, such as surveys to gauge family workers' expertise and gain knowledge about their relatives and the care they needed.

Organisational documents do not reflect family workers' labour or involvement. Nor do they outline actual institutional processes or details on safe work environments for family workers. On the one hand, flexible documentation and job descriptions can provide flexibility in interpreting regulations. On the other, the absence of family workers in these documents and procedures underscores the invisibility of family workers' work, despite how necessary it is for the care of residents.

Conditions of work and care

Given the high amount of unpaid work that family workers undertake, interactions with other paid workers in nursing homes are important. Our research shows that recognising and supporting family workers' involvement involves supporting staff and their conditions of work.

Family and staff perceptions of family work

Family workers may want to be involved in some forms of care work in nursing homes, and the ability to engage in meaningful activities and relationships should be available for families, along with appropriate support. Other forms of care work are burdensome and may leave family workers with little time to do other things. Some family workers enjoy providing unpaid work and care, while others find it oppressive and see it as a generative cycle for women and caring. Some family workers told us how grateful they were to be relieved of caring for their loved one. This raises the question of whether or not the work is rewarding or burdensome, whether it's done by choice or compulsion, and how to protect families doing this work.

Many staff said they welcomed the support from family workers and paid companions, because of their poor working conditions. Echoing Gaugler's research (2005), one staff member explained, "Unfortunately ... you know, with the time constraints, family help is ... welcomed". Workers talked about their interactions with families and their sometimes close relationships with them, giving us examples of situations that were not represented in the organisational documents. For example, personal support workers (PSWs) described the physical work they did with residents and families:

'[F]amily coming to pick up a resident to take them out, right in the front of the door, you can see that they're struggling with a resident to properly lift them and get them into a car, so we would go and offer help and you could see banging on a window. If we get injured out there, we're not covered.' (Interview with PSW)

The same PSW talked about their deep involvement with family workers in the home: "Some families − we'll cry with some of the family members." Yet the organisational documents offered no indication of PSWs interacting with families.

Putting family workers' rights and protections on the agenda

Canadian staff are facing low staff to patient ratios, higher resident acuity levels, and increasing reporting requirements (Armstrong et al, 2009; Daly et al, 2015). New public management (NPM), introduced by neoliberal governments to reduce the costs of care, has a strong impact on work organisation (Armstrong and Braedley, 2013), including by stipulating reporting requirements that aim to ensure accountability and efficiencies (Baines and Cunningham, 2013; Daly, 2015). Meanwhile, structural barriers mean workers tend to prioritise residents' physical care before social care (Barken and Lowndes, 2017). A focus on physical and medical tasks too often leaves the social support to be provided without pay. But staff do not have the time to complete basic tasks in current job descriptions, let alone attend to complex and necessary coordination with family workers. Feminist political economists have found that despite NPM's claims to advance the quality of care and improve practices, it in fact increases pace and workload, decreases the time for social care, and shifts responsibilities for care to individuals at home (Baines and Armstrong, 2018).

Family workers often make links between their own involvement and staffing shortages and underfunding. Unpaid family workers partially cover absences and deficits in paid care work. The wife of an ex-husband who's in a nursing home explained how she stepped in to help to physically lift her husband when workers were too busy, as he is "not supposed to be put into bed without two people". She also said that, with how "busy people are", some family workers think, "Well, I'll just do it quick", which puts them at risk of hurting themselves.

This type of unpaid work could cause harm to family workers and can create distrust between staff and family/friends (Ryan and Scullion, 2000; Holmgren et al, 2012). It also encourages the nursing home's reliance on these individuals to provide this care. One participant described the predicament that she put herself in by participating in this type of unpaid work: "[A]s I say, I've created somewhat of a monster, because they know I will be here. So often they don't even come and check in the room. 'Well, his wife is there. We don't need to take him to choir or bingo or anything else'."

Staff commented on their frequent double shifts, the lack of time for proper care, and the unacceptable ratios in daily care. As one director of care put it, "There's just not enough time. … It's just absolutely unacceptable the time that people get". Many noted that working short was often "when mistakes happen" which they would be "held liable for". With appropriate staffing levels and hours, staff would have sufficient time to provide care as well as interact with family workers who were also providing care (Baumbusch and Phinney, 2013). Recognising and supporting family workers' involvement requires supporting staff and their conditions of work.

Promising practices and a politicised conception of family work

A central assumption in our research is that the conditions of work are the conditions of care. This chapter uses the term 'family workers' to orient their unpaid work of family/friends as a form of work that requires adequate conditions and protections. Viewing family/friends as workers acknowledges that some family workers' contributions are essential to the operation of a nursing home. The point is that this term could be used in document processes and policies to recognise and acknowledge the skilled work that families are contributing and to provide the needed protections and conditions for their work (Armstrong, 2013). Importantly, recognising and supporting family workers' involvement also involves supporting staff and their conditions of work.

Establishing some promising practices for family workers is particularly important because administrators and paid workers are already stretched too thinly and don't have time to figure out how or when to include family workers in work processes. Teamwork, communication, spaces and locations are all important considerations when it comes to improving the working conditions of family workers (Barken and Lowndes, 2017). Families also need both a physically safe work environment, like that recommended by the World Health Organization (WHO, 2007), and a psychologically safe work environment, especially in light of the pandemic (Shain, 2010).

Paid workers in nursing homes need these improvements as well (Braedley et al, 2017). Unions provide staff with these important rights and protections, despite limited funding. Workers' rights and protections are important, and unpaid family workers should have them too. Family workers should be included in more specific ways within policies and procedures set out in nursing home documents. They should be included in the creation of procedures for coordination between them and staff. This collaboration, however, is not imaginable without adequate staffing, time and support for paid staff (Austin et al, 2009). Proper time and resources for collaboration and coordination between staff and family workers to articulate these working conditions in documents have the potential to improve care to residents.

We found promising practices for the recognition of family workers in these nursing homes that, if given time and resources, could improve conditions of work and conditions of care. Promising articulations of the role of family workers were often found in the work of the family councils. One family worker explained how the family council worked to raise money for the nursing home for important improvements in the home. Another family council was described as "very active" in working towards improving experiences at the nursing home. And in light of the challenges caused by the pandemic, family councils increased their efforts on advocacy, staff shortages, national standards and improved capacity, not to mention the numerous education events they sponsored to share information and ideas.

I hope my analysis helps foster solidarity between family workers and paid workers to advocate for and support each other in improving working conditions and in developing an enriched care environment for everyone. The term 'solidarity' emphasises the already evident connection between paid and unpaid workers, who have a mutual commitment to care for residents (Laitinen and Pessi, 2014). Solidarity is a relational strategy where paid and unpaid workers can work together to promote changes in the areas of their shared concerns, and to challenge limiting neoliberal strategies (Baines and Daly, 2019).

Improving the conditions of care for both staff and family workers

Our research helps make visible the multiple forms of family workers' unpaid work, such as personalising, coordinating and advocating for care. The encounter between the family worker and paid staff is rarely articulated in terms of labour processes, and often families' work is lacking the appropriate working conditions because of the invisibility of the work. Organisational documents that focus on communication with family/friends do not account for family workers' contributions; nor do they reflect a nursing home's dependence and reliance on family workers' unpaid work (Barken et al, 2016). This chapter found a narrow specification for family workers' work, extensive staff involvement with family workers, and a lack of physical and psychological safety protections for family workers, reinforcing the undervaluing of their skills and contributions. Family councils are central to improving support and advocacy.

Our research shows that for the most part, paid workers welcomed family workers' support under challenging working conditions. We establish the political importance of adequate staffing, which would increase the practical time and support available for paid staff to collaborate with family workers while recognising their work and improving work processes and dynamics. In the face of pandemic challenges, labour shortages and inadequate public services, further reflection on work and staff–family interactions would clearly support initiatives to foster solidarity and develop enriched care environments for everyone.

Notes

[1]   The concept of 'family' used here includes spouses or adult children, but also 'chosen family' and close friends who are responsible for unpaid care work, or alternative family forms, such as ones that are more common for lesbian, gay, bisexual, transgender, or queer (LGBTQ) folks (Brotman and Ferrer, 2015).

[2]   Documents included resident care manuals/handbooks, job descriptions, primary care assignments, employee handbooks and organisational documents such as quality improvement plans, strategic plans and annual reports.

References

Armstrong, P. (2013) Puzzling skills: Feminist political economy approaches, *Canadian Review of Sociology/Revue canadienne de sociologie*, 50(3): 256–83, https://doi.org/10.1111/cars.12015

Armstrong, P., Banerjee, A., Szebehely, M. and Armstrong, H. (2009) *They Deserve Better: The Long-term Care Experience in Canada and Scandinavia*, Canadian Centre for Policy Alternatives.

Armstrong, P. and Braedley, S. (eds) (2013) *Troubling Care: Critical Perspectives on Research and Practices*, Canadian Scholars Press.

Armstrong, P. and Day, S. (2020) Clothing matters: Locating wash, wear, and care, *Studies in Political Economy*, 101(1): 1–16, https://doi.org/10.1080/07078552.2020.1738777

Armstrong, P. and Lowndes, R. (eds) (2018) *Creative Teamwork: Developing Rapid, Site-switching Ethnography*, Oxford University Press.

Austin, W., Goble, E., Strang, V., Mitchell, A., Thompson, E., Lantz, H., Balt, L., Lemermeyer, G. and Vass, K. (2009) Supporting relationships between family and staff in continuing care settings, *Journal of Family Nursing*, 15(3): 360–83, https://doi.org/10.1177/1074840709339781

Baines, D. and Armstrong, P. (2018) Non-job work/unpaid caring: Gendered industrial relations in long-term care, *Gender, Work & Organization*, 26(7): 934–47, https://doi.org/10.1111/gwao.12293

Baines, D. and Cunningham, I. (2013) Using comparative perspective rapid ethnography in international case studies, *Qualitative Social Work*, 12: 73–88.

Baines, D. and Daly, T. (2019) Borrowed time and solidarity: The multi-scalar politics of time and gendered care work, *Social Politics: International Studies in Gender, State & Society*, 28(2): 385–404, https://doi.org/10.1093/sp/jxz017

Barken, R., Daly, T.J. and Armstrong, P. (2016) Family matters: The work and skills of family/friend carers in long-term residential care, *Journal of Canadian Studies*, 50(2): 321–47, https://doi.org/10.3138/jcs.50.2.321

Barken, R. and Lowndes, R. (2017) Supporting family involvement in long-term residential care: Promising practices for relational care, *Qualitative Health Research*, 28(1): 60–72, https://doi.org/10.1177/10497 32317730568

Baumbusch, J. and Phinney, A. (2013) Invisible hands, *Journal of Family Nursing*, 20(1): 73–97, https://doi.org/10.1177/1074840713507777

Braedley, S., Owusu, P., Przednowek, A. and Armstrong, P. (2017) We're told, 'suck it up': Long-term care workers' psychological health and safety, *Ageing International*, 43(1): 91–109, https://doi.org/10.1007/s12 126-017-9288-4

Bowen, G.A. (2009) Document analysis as a qualitative research method, *Qualitative Research Journal*, 9(2): 27–40, doi:10.3316/QRJ0902027

Brotman, S. and Ferrer, I. (2015) Diversity within family caregiving: Extending definitions of 'who counts' to include marginalized communities, *Healthcare Papers*, 15(1): 47–53, https://doi.org/10.12927/hcpap.2015.24395

Change Foundation (2016) *Enhancing Care, Enhancing Life: Impacts of Residents' Councils and Family Councils in Ontario Long Term Care Homes*, The Change Foundation, pp 1–36. https://fco.ngo/news/enhancing-care-enhancing-life-reflections-on-the-change-foundation-report

Daly, T. (2015) Dancing the two-step in Ontario's long term care sector: Deterrence regulation = consolidation, *Studies in Political Economy*, 95(1): 29–58.

Daly, T., Armstrong, P. and Lowndes, R. (2015) Liminality in Ontario's long-term care facilities: Private companions' care work in the space "betwixt and between", *Competition & Change*, 19(3): 246–63, https://doi.org/10.1177/1024529415580262

England, P., Budig, M. and Folbre, N. (2002) Wages of virtue: The relative pay of care work, *Social Problems*, 49(4): 455–73.

Family Councils ON (nd) 'Family Councils 101', Available from: http://fco.ngo/https://fco.ngo/resources/family-councils-101

Gaugler, J.E. (2005) Family involvement in residential long-term care: A synthesis and critical review, *Aging & Mental Health*, 9(2): 105–18, https://doi.org/10.1080/13607860412331310245

Gladstone, J.W., Dupuis, S.L. and Wexler, E. (2006) Changes in family involvement following a relative's move to a long-term care facility, *Canadian Journal on Aging/La Revue canadienne du vieillissement*, 25(1): 93–106, https://doi.org/10.1353/cja.2006.0022

Holmgren, J., Emami, A., Eriksson, L.E. and Eriksson, H. (2012) Being perceived as a 'visitor' in the nursing staff's working arena: The involvement of relatives in daily caring activities in nursing homes in an urban community in Sweden, *Scandinavian Journal of Caring Sciences*, 27(3): 677–85, https://doi.org/10.1111/j.1471-6712.2012.01077.x

Koren, M.J. (2010) Person-centered care for nursing home residents: The culture-change movement, *Health Affairs*, 29(2): 312–17, https://doi.org/ten.1377/hlthaff.2009.0966

Laitinen, A. and Pessi, A.B. (2014) *Solidarity: Theory and Practice*, Lexington Books.

Luxton, M. (2006) Feminist political economy in Canada and the politics of social reproduction, in K. Bezanson and M. Luxton (eds) *Social Reproduction: Feminist Political Economy Challenges Neoliberalism*, McGill-Queen's University Press, pp 11–44.

O'Leary, Z. (2014) *The Essential Guide to Doing Your Research Project* (2nd edn), SAGE Publications, Inc.

Ryan, A.A. and Scullion, H. F. (2000) Family and staff perceptions of the role of families in nursing homes, *Journal of Advanced Nursing*, 32(3): 626–34, https://doi.org/10.1046/j.1365-2648.2000.01521.x

Shain, M. (2010) *Tracking the Perfect Legal Storm*, Mental Health Commission of Canada.

World Health Organization (WHO) (2007) *Workers' Health: Global Plan of Action*, 6th World Health Assembly.

7

Staff perspectives on families' unpaid work in care homes

Ruth Lowndes, Marta Szebehely, Gudmund Ågotnes and Oddrunn Sortland

In this chapter we compare and analyse relationships between staff and the families of residents in Canadian, Norwegian and Swedish care homes. As we know from Chapter 1, care homes differ considerably in size, staffing levels and organisation of the daily work. These contextual differences shape the scope and need for families' unpaid work and how families are perceived by staff. We base our analysis on 65 interviews conducted between 2018 and 2019 with frontline staff and managers and on fieldnotes from studying eight care homes.

The models of care in the three jurisdictions vary from social care models we observed in Sweden to medical models of care we observed in Canada and to a lesser degree in Norway (Ågotnes et al, 2017; Szebehely, 2017). Work is conceptualised and organised differently within these models (Day, 2013). In contrast to social care models, in which care relationships are central, in medical care approaches, biomedical needs are emphasised while the relational aspects of care are not given high priority (Day, 2013). In addition, low staffing levels within the Canadian context impact staff's ability to form relationships with residents and families (Lowndes and Struthers, 2018). These differences affect the boundaries between the care work carried out by staff, families and friends, leading to varying boundaries between paid and unpaid work in the three countries.

Research on unpaid care work provided by families and friends does not often concern itself with what happens inside the care homes, even though it is clear that family members continue to provide care after their relative is admitted (Ryan and Scullion, 2000b). Roles, tasks and relationships with relatives, other residents and staff change over time and place. Clearly, it is beneficial for both staff and family carers to have well-functioning, stable relationships, and to work together to improve residents' quality of life (Pillemer et al, 1998; Ward-Griffin et al, 2003; Bauer, 2006; McGilton and Boscart, 2007). More information is needed on factors that influence the development, or lack of development, of relationships between staff and families (Ward-Griffin et al, 2003), and on policies and practices that include families in care provision in meaningful ways (Barken and Lowndes, 2018).

The research we have indicates tensions and differing boundaries. As the Ryan and Scullion (2000a) study in rural Northern Ireland suggests, staff may not trust families to carry out care work, especially tasks involving certain risks, such as lifting, and may underestimate the value of family involvement in care. The Swedish study carried out by Hertzberg et al (2003) also found that staff viewed families as a resource for their relative's well-being because of their visits and the information they provided, but preferred that family members not be involved in 'too much hands-on care' (p 440).

An Australian study (Bauer, 2007) also indicated that staff wanted to retain control of the workplace and 'preferred families to confine themselves to non-care giving activities and roles which were free of risks, and which did not hold up the work that staff did' (p 215). Staff also found that some family behaviours reflected limited understanding of resident care and the realities of care work in these settings (Bauer, 2007). For instance, 'demanding' families made frequent requests and expected immediate attention, interfering with care work that had to be completed in a restricted timeframe (Bauer, 2007). Other researchers, such as Utley-Smith and colleagues (2009) and Sortland (2020), have documented how staff may perceive interaction with families as challenging and time-consuming, and may also describe some families as 'demanding'.

Different physical environments and staffing conditions

The eight care homes that form the basis for our analysis vary in size, organisation, and staffing. In Ontario, Canada, the three homes ranged in size from 112 to 450 beds, with both semi-private and private bedrooms in units accommodating anywhere from 20 to 32 residents. In Sweden, one home had 57 apartments divided into four units, and the other had 36 apartments divided into four units. As is typical in Sweden, all residents had private apartments with a bathroom, a kitchenette and usually a private balcony. In Norway, one rural home had 50 beds, all in private rooms, with some residents sharing a bathroom. The other rural home in Norway had 56 private rooms with private bathrooms organised into six units, while the urban home had seven units with a total of 107 private rooms with bathrooms.

The data in Chapter 1 showing much higher staffing levels in Scandinavian care homes are reflected in the homes of this study. The Ontario homes were much bigger than the Scandinavian homes and also the units were bigger, with around 30 residents in each unit. Typically, there were at least nine residents per worker during a dayshift. Staff told us they often worked in short-staffed situations. In the biggest Ontario home, with 450 residents, staffing ratios were similar, except in the dedicated veterans' units, owing to extra funding from Veterans Affairs Canada. The Swedish and Norwegian homes included in the study had much higher staffing levels, with three to four residents per worker on a dayshift during the week. There was also a much higher presence of registered nurses (RNs) in the Norwegian homes than in the homes in both Sweden and Ontario.

Different frameworks for families

The three jurisdictions varied in their formal policies and procedures for families visiting care homes. In the Swedish homes, each resident had a contact person, who was responsible for following up on one or two residents, including communicating with their families. The contact person made and updated the resident's care plan, and had extra responsibility for the resident's personal care and for providing them with practical help, including assisting with cleaning and laundry. The same care worker normally remained the primary contact throughout the resident's stay.

This worker was expected to establish contact and build trust with the family. One assistant nurse explained, "I have the main responsibility to create a relationship with the family and with residents also, of course". Another said, "They can turn to me if there is something they are worried about or want help with. And I have to make sure how things are with them, how they are doing".

The Norwegian homes also had this system, which staff considered important: "As primary contact I am responsible for contacting family if the residents need anything, [for instance] clothes, or they have birthdays; then we call them if they need a cake, or [if there is] anything they need for their rooms" (assistant nurse, Norway). Another Norwegian assistant nurse agreed on the importance of having a contact person, but, in contrast to the Swedish care workers, emphasised medical tasks, reflecting a stronger medical focus in Norwegian homes:

> 'When we have a primary contact, the follow-up is much better. Better than just having a written plan – not everybody follows that, and not everybody tidies the room even. So having more responsibility is better. We even monitor their weight and their blood pressure, how much they eat. So not only clothes, but much more medical. We have one or two each.'

Although one Ontario site had a primary nurse and another assigned primary personal support worker (PSW) unlike in Scandinavia, the nurses and PSWs did not commonly have responsibility for contacting particular residents' families. The RNs and RPNs (registered practical nurses) in Ontario were usually responsible for relaying any medical information to family members, while the PSWs provided most of the hands-on care. There were no specific guidelines for connecting with families, but if family wanted to be involved, staff stressed that their role should be documented in the resident's care plan. At the same time, staffing shortages and reliance on part-time and casual staff negatively affected care continuity in Ontario.

Different family work roles

In all three jurisdictions, families were generally viewed positively and as crucial for the well-being of residents. In the Swedish homes, families were considered to be important as *visitors* for the residents, to provide needed socialisation, and to *bring knowledge* and insights about their relative. They were not expected or encouraged to do practical work for the resident: "It's very important for staff, residents, family that we can trust each other and feel safe with each other. Otherwise, it doesn't work, we can't work without family. They provide images. They know their relatives. You can't take them away. We need them" (Interview with assistant nurse, Sweden).

Similarly, in Norway, families were expected to spend time socialising with residents, rather than doing unpaid work. However, unlike in Sweden, families were expected to take the resident on outings and to medical appointments. An RN in a Norwegian home explained: "They visit. And we do the rest. And sometimes go out, but they could do more of that." A manager in another Norwegian home reported:

'We don't expect the families to provide practical help to the care home, but we expect them to help their family member – for example, taking them to the hospital for appointments, buying clothes and shoes, showing interest for their well-being and engaging in arrangements in the care home if possible.'

So families in Norwegian homes are expected to do some unpaid work for the resident, a message much less heard in the Swedish homes.

In the Ontario sites, where staffing levels were low, families were welcome and often expected to fill the care gaps. As an Ontario director of care explained, "Unfortunately, you know, with time constraints ... family help is welcomed". Family members' work in these homes often involved tasks like cleaning their relatives' room, doing laundry, shopping and arranging for and accompanying them to medical appointments. Staff had very little time to spend talking to residents or taking them outside for fresh air, so family social care was critical. The expected amount of unpaid work could be extensive. Here's what the director of care in one home said:

> 'We encourage family participation in care. … So, if the husband or daughter wants to participate in the bath, sometimes it's beneficial because we have the behaviours of people with dementia of various sorts where they're the only ones that are able to bathe. We would care plan that, but first the registered staff would assess that they're safely able to do the activity that they're wanting to do.'

Family members in the Ontario sites were often involved in assisting residents with eating: "A lot of families [come and help]. There are some families that come every single day" (Interview with resident and family services supervisor, Ontario). Family members' help was appreciated, as an RPN made clear: "I find when family members come and they'll brush the family members' teeth or help them get their clothes on for bed … just different things like that, small things just to help support the PSWs because they have a really busy job."

None of the staff interviewed in the Scandinavian homes mentioned personal care as a task that families did or were expected to do. Higher staffing levels made this kind of unpaid work less necessary. It was also seen as crucial for the dignity and integrity of the resident to receive such help from trained workers, rather than from family members, reflecting the way 'care work' is embedded with a notion of professional skill in a Scandinavian context. A recent Swedish care home study showed that families and staff shared this sentiment: families preferred to leave bodily care to care workers, having confidence that they had the skills (and time) needed to provide intimate care in a competent way (Holmberg et al, 2020).

The first encounter between staff and families

In the Swedish homes, the first encounter between staff and family was considered paramount in establishing a solid rapport, building trust and avoiding future difficulties: "The first time here is so important, and the first meeting. … That's the first stone [brick] we are building" (Interview with care aide, Sweden). Another staff member stressed the importance of a warm welcome: "It is extremely important that they get a first positive impression. That's 99 per cent of the base for building a good relationship. If they get a bad impression, then it's hopeless. It's over. Then it's very difficult to build a good relationship" (Interview with assistant nurse, Sweden).

In the Norwegian and Ontario homes, the admission process was time-constrained. A rush to fill the bed impacted the first encounter. In Norway, this meant that the first meeting with new residents and family members was difficult to schedule:

'When they know about an opening, the families often come to have a look at the rooms beforehand. How long before varies, usually some days before. It happens after a death, because we are full. So, when someone dies, a room is available. It usually doesn't take long, but it depends. We have meetings once a week, so it depends on the meeting. And, of course, it depends on whether the family is ready or not.' (Interview with RN, Norway)

While Sweden has a standard system for the first encounter, this was not the case in the Norwegian homes. One Norwegian home had tried to have regular 'intake meetings' with the resident, family and physician, but had to give it up because the physician did not have the time. However, staff saw the benefit of an organised first meeting: "If we have an early meeting where we can clarify expectations and have a realistic conversation about the situation and tell them how things work here, then the communication works much better later on" (Interview with RN, Norway).

In Ontario, the resident and family have 24 hours to decide if they will take the bed when it becomes available (OLTCA, 2021), and only five days to complete the move (see Chapter 2). Recognising that the admission process was overwhelming for families, one Ontario site had recently added an RPN position in the Admissions Office: "So [that] anything that could be done with the family or resident, if competent, is done before the day they get here" (Interview with director of nursing, Ontario). In another home, a staff member explained: "I love to talk to the family and just put them at ease too because it's very intimidating the first day moving here or to special care" (Interview with resident special program coordinator, Ontario). In a third home, an RN explained how circumstances differed between residents:

'I think it depends on the resident. And if there's family involvement and that sort of thing, because sometimes they're just dragged and dropped. ... Sometimes, there might be a family member to come and sign some paperwork and then they leave, and it's like OK, well, if that resident can't tell us their routine, we fly by the seat of our pants and we really, really hope that that resident wants to be here because if they don't, then it makes it ten times harder to figure out how we're going to make this work with this scared resident that's brand new, doesn't know the building and has no support system.'

The admission process can be overwhelming especially when rushed, as in Norway and Ontario. The deliberate emphasis on first contact as the starting point for relationship building, coupled with one staff member being the main contact for each resident throughout their stay, developed trusting relationships.

Increased presence of families

In all the care homes we studied, residents made the move into a home late in life and were frail with multiple co-morbidities. In all three countries, there is an increasing complexity of resident needs due to a reduced number of care home beds and more stringent criteria for admission. Staffing levels in care homes have not kept pace with these changes. Consequently, families, especially in Ontario, are often more involved in what could be considered fundamental unpaid work. At the same time, families' expectations have changed. A staff member described the difference over time:

> 'Well, they're always trying to do more with less, you know. Back in the old days, residents were just sort of put in a home and forgotten many of them, and now we're seeing more involved families. We're dealing with very demanding family members as well as demanding residents too.' (Interview with RPN, Ontario)

In the Swedish sites, families were similarly more involved now than previously. This was partly related to feeling welcomed as visitors, but also to being more informed about their rights and more worried, given negative media reports. This sentiment was echoed in the following exchange:

Interviewer: Has the relation to family changed during the years you have been working?
Respondent: No, not really. Maybe [it's] a bit more active, maybe [they] make more visits.
Interviewer: Why?
Respondent: In the beginning they might be worried, they are on guard, have got their view on eldercare from media, and that's not a positive image. But we can change their mind quickly. … They know their rights more than earlier. They know that they have the right to a contact person.
                                (Interview with assistant nurse, Sweden)

Similarly, in Norway, staff described more engaged and active family members. Staff described families' greater awareness of and knowledge about rights, and how the homes facilitated family involvement, trying out new avenues:

> 'They ask about what happens at this place, what they can be part of. Before, when this was an 'older people's home' and not a nursing home, there wasn't much happening. They just sat there. But we have

tried to change this. We also use Facebook for this. All families have access to this, and they have to sign a form if their family members can be pictured there. And then they can follow what's happening, to stay updated. They get reassured.' (Interview with manager, Norway)

In all three countries, we were told that families were more involved in their relatives' care and better informed about the residents' rights than in the past. One reason could be that the homes were more actively inviting families to visit the homes. However, the increased presence of families could also be related to staff shortages, especially in the Ontario context, where families often felt the need to continue caring for increasingly frail relatives in the nursing home.

Handling tensions with families

Instances of conflicts between family and staff were described in all the care homes. Common family complaints in the Ontario homes included missing or damaged laundry, poor teeth cleaning and items stolen from residents. Staff described some families as "challenging" or "squeaky". Some were described as having unrealistic expectations: "The families are in denial of how confused or demented the resident is" (Interview with RPN, Ontario). Staff also reported that sometimes families needed to be educated. For example, during one site visit, a care home was removing bedrails because of entrapment concerns, and staff said that family members who were advocating to keep them needed to learn about the use of restraints.

Tensions in family dynamics were recognised as requiring negotiation: "Siblings don't get along and disagree with the treatment" (RPN, Ontario). These tensions were also reported in the Scandinavian homes, according to a manager in Norway:

'We had a very ill resident who had a lot of children. Many were involved and everybody had an opinion, different opinion, so we spent a lot of time on this family, and it affected other residents. Every time somebody came, they wanted information and they grabbed some of the staff to ask. And in the end, we had to sit down and have a meeting, and I said they needed to agree on *one* of them to gather and ask questions and get information. *I* should answer all the questions.' (Manager, Norway)

In all three jurisdictions, staff and management reported struggles with tensions and with attempts to balance family and resident needs. In the Ontario homes, where staff were responsible for many residents, and had heavy workloads and competing demands, care workers described concerns that families did not recognise the amount of work staff had to do: "They're all under the impression that there's not 28 residents. There's my mom. And I want my mom taken care of. I don't care about anybody else. It's like, but there are 27 other residents" (PSW, Ontario). In the Scandinavian sites, where staffing levels were much higher, this issue was less frequently reported but not entirely absent. As one Norwegian assistant nurse told us: "Sometimes you feel they [families] have to see the other residents. Don't just look at your own relative. They don't see all the others that need help too."

A more frequent tension reported in the Swedish and Norwegian sites was that staff and families often had differing viewpoints on resident needs. In situations where negotiation was required, staff generally supported residents over families to ensure their needs were met:

> 'Sometimes they say "This is how Mum wants it"', and we know, we have tried, and we know that she doesn't really want it that way. After all, it's we who are there helping. We can listen to what they say and have it in mind, but in the end we do it the way the resident wants. … It usually gets resolved if you have an open dialogue and are honest – 'I hear what you say, but we want them to be well' – then they feel safe. They are insecure when the resident moves in, [not knowing] what kind of place this is – "Are you [going] to take care of my mum?"' (Interview with assistant nurse, Sweden)

Staff described various ways of handling problematic situations with families. In the Swedish homes, the first meeting with the resident and family was regarded as crucial to avoid future difficulties: "It's very important, it's not about handing out some papers in a fast way. It is a very important meeting – building trust, that they can call whenever they have any questions" (Group leader, Sweden).

This proactive strategy to build relationships as a means of avoiding problems in the future, as well as the contact person's role, was stressed by both managers and care workers in the Swedish homes. In all three of the Ontario sites, leaders emphasised the importance of being accessible. One manager reported being available 24/7 via cell phone to avoid escalation of an issue. "Sometimes we have very squeaky families … and sometimes it's better for me to take a squeaky family phone call at 7 pm than it is for me to wait until the next day."

Some Ontario staff described feeling unsupported when family conflicts arose. As an RPN put it: "We're not supported. I do not believe we are supported one bit … they take it all out on you, they go to management and that's it." Another RPN described how she was reprimanded for acceding to a family member's urgent request to pick her up and drive her to the care home when her father, a resident of six years, was not doing well: "Sometimes you think quicker with your heart than you do with your brain, and it sometimes bites you."

A manager in another Ontario home described accommodating families who, for various reasons, didn't want specific staff caring for their relative:

'Recently on one of my units a high-needs family didn't want certain caregivers, certain PSWs, taking care of their loved one. And we are more than willing to make that accommodation. ... A really tough conversation to have with PSWs, to say that to somebody, especially when I know that they give good care. But ... the family can't see that, and they just don't want that PSW in that room with their dad.' (Manager, Ontario)

We also heard about tensions with family members in the Scandinavian sites. In Norway, complaints were often connected to the perceived deterioration of residents, which sometimes led to family members blaming staff for not doing enough:

'We hear that they have too few clothes on in the winter, stuff like that. Perhaps someone feels that their father has deteriorated so much lately, and that it is because we have not exercised enough with him. We have put in a great effort, but perhaps they haven't noticed. Especially with one. Last time I talked to her, she started, the daughter, and she said that we do not train [exercise them] enough. I said that we have tried, in a nice way. In the end she said, "Well, well, she is getting older", so perhaps she has changed. But I believe that it is the manager who gets most of it.' (RN, Norway)

Other staff members in the Scandinavian sites reported that managers usually took care of family members who presented challenges, and that the staff rarely felt lack of support from management. In one Swedish home, a manager met with the daughter of a resident who complained and made racist comments. She sat with the daughter once a week for an entire year in order to support staff.

'In the end it became unsustainable, so I contacted her and said, "We have to sit down together". So we sat together one evening, from 6 to 9 and sorted it out. I said, "I can't have it this way". She had some relevant criticism, but then she started to say [about a worker], "She is fat and lazy and sits on her bum", and I said, "You have *nothing* to do with what my staff look like or what skin colour they have!" But we agreed to meet once a week. I said, "It's better that you come to me and talk about what you think, then I can act and you can get an explanation about things we can't do anything about, and other things I can bring to the staff". And for a year she came once a week, and then every second week. And sometimes she just came by and said hello. I felt it was necessary to do it this way, to rescue the staff and also my own work environment.' (Manager, Sweden)

This manager stressed that "You have to consider the relative's situation, but you must also consider the staff's work environment".

Context matters!

In this study, we found that overall, staff had positive perceptions of families. However, different contextual conditions shaped the various roles that families navigated alongside and with staff, and the amount and form of unpaid work they carried out in the home. These conditions also shaped the types and depth of relationships that formed between staff and families. Such factors as having a contact-person model, small units and high staffing levels left room and space for closer social connections and continuity between residents, family and staff. Together with more scope for managerial support when family conflicts arose, an emphasis on social care impacted staff perceptions of families, and if and how family members were involved in day-to-day life at the care home.

Staffing levels were critical in determining the amount and type of work families carried out. Families in the Scandinavian homes were not required to fill in care gaps; rather they were viewed as visitors who provided social support. Higher staffing levels also provided opportunities such as extra time for staff to build relationships with families and for managers to support staff and families. This contrasted with what we observed in the Ontario sites, where the much lower staffing levels meant families were encouraged to do extensive amounts of work to fill the care gap caused by underfunding.

In all three jurisdictions, residents are entering long-term care at later stages in life and with complex co-morbidities. However, the low staffing levels in Ontario, which have not kept up with the increasing frailty of resident populations, particularly in for-profit homes (McGregor and Ronald, 2011), result in heavy workloads and in staff juggling competing demands, a finding echoed in the literature (McGilton and Boscart, 2007; Majerovitz et al, 2009). Staff have little time under these conditions to engage in good communication (Majerovitz et al, 2009) and build meaningful relationships.

Furthermore, Ontario operates within a highly medicalised, task-oriented model of care, where biomedical needs are prioritised. We, along with Bauer (2006, p 51), argue that an environment where relational and social needs and care are secondary is not family-friendly. Although Norwegian homes are more medicalised than the Swedish sites we studied, social care is prioritised to a greater degree than what we found in Ontario. This is reflected in smaller, homelike units with fewer residents, which facilitates continuity of care and the building of relationships. In the Swedish sites, social care is explicitly emphasised: work is not task-oriented, and staff are afforded time to engage with residents and families, and to build relationships with them. However, care workers in Sweden also experienced time pressures, because there too, staffing has not kept pace with increasing care needs, leaving the workers with more physical and mental fatigue than previously, and with increasing intentions to quit (Stranz and Szebehely, 2018).

Although families were generally viewed positively by staff in our study, and staff expressed the importance of family involvement, all sites reported encountering difficult family interactions. Staff reported that some families did not understand the work pressures, such as time constraints and heavy workloads. Some family members wanted immediate attention and some families were problematic, demanding attention and hard to please, just as Utley-Smith and colleagues (2009) found. These families were viewed as time-consuming and difficult. Staff described the same concerns as Bauer (2007) reported: some families lacked insight, sometimes interfered with care, or made demands and could not be satisfied, and we too, found that "familial disputes at times manifested in the nursing home" (p 216). Staff described instances of conflict within a family where they felt they were put into the middle and had to manage the tensions.

The literature on staff and family relationships emphasises the importance of admission as a starting point to the process of providing information, orienting families to the care home, and letting them know that their ongoing support and advocacy are appreciated (Majerovitz et al, 2009). Ontario's admission process is rushed, with restricted time to accept a bed, move in and complete necessary paperwork, and it can be overwhelming for all concerned (Chapter 2). An RPN position that was added in one home to assist with the admission process – with the goal of having as much done as possible before the actual move-in day – helped reduce tensions. The fact that the RPN reached out to gather information and to answer questions also helped to initiate communication with families.

The Norwegian staff facilitated a welcoming atmosphere when meeting families and residents for the first time. But because residents arrive within two or three days of a room becoming available, the process was not always thoroughly planned and was dependent on the situation in the unit on that particular day. Uncertainty and misunderstandings between families and staff might result. In the Swedish homes, the admission was viewed by management and staff as an opportunity both to initiate contact and to begin building trusting relationships, thereby avoiding potential conflicts later. To support families in choosing what work they want to do for their relatives and to avoid tensions between staff and families, we found a deliberate introductory process and a contact person model to be promising practices. However, these systems are not achievable without sufficient staffing levels and support from management. Without them, there will continue to be tensions between staff and families and demands on both families and staff to bridge care gaps with unpaid work.

References

Ågotnes, G., Jacobsen, F.F. and Barken, R. (2017) A Norwegian view on Canadian long-term residential care, *Journal of Canadian Studies*, 50(2): 491–98.

Barken, R. and Lowndes, R. (2018) Supporting family involvement in long-term residential care: Promising practices for relational care, *Qualitative Health Research*, 28(1): 60–72.

Bauer, M. (2006) Collaboration and control: Nurses' constructions of the role of family in nursing home care, *Journal of Advanced Nursing*, 54(1): 45–52.

Bauer, M. (2007) Staff-family relationships in nursing home care: A typology of challenging behaviours, *International Journal of Older People Nursing*, 2: 213–18.

Day, S. (2013) The implications of conceptualizing care, in P. Armstrong and S. Braedley (eds) *Troubling Care: Critical Perspectives on Research and Practices*, Canadian Scholar's Press, pp 21–32.

Hertzberg, A., Ekman, S. and Axelsson, K. (2003) 'Relatives are a resource, but … ': Registered nurses' views and experiences of relatives of residents in nursing homes, *Journal of Clinical Nursing*, 12: 431–41.

Holmberg, B., Hellström, I. and Österlind, J. (2020) Being a spectator in ambiguity: Family members' perceptions of assisted bodily care in a nursing home, *International Journal of Older People Nursing*, 15(1): e12289, doi:10.1111/opn.12289

Lowndes, R. and Struthers, J. (2018) A day in the life: Comparisons of medical and social care models in Germany and Ontario, in P. Armstrong and R. Lowndes (eds) *Negotiating Tensions in Long-term Residential Care: Ideas Worth Sharing*, Canadian Centre for Policy Alternatives, pp 67–74.

Majerovitz, S.D., Mollott, R. and Rudder, C. (2009) We're on the same side: Improving communication between nursing home and family, *Health Communication*, 24: 12–20.

McGilton, K. and Boscart, V. (2007) Close care provider-resident relationships in long-term care environments, *Journal of Clinical Nursing*, 16: 2149–57.

McGregor, M. and Ronald, L. (2011) Residential long-term care for Canadian seniors: Nonprofit, for-profit, or does it matter? IRPP Study No. 14, Available from: https://irpp.org/wp-content/uploads/2011/01/study-no14.pdf

Ontario Long-term Care Association (OLTCA) (2021) 'The role of long-term care', Available from: https://www.oltca.com/oltca/OLTCA/Public/LongTermCare/FactsFigures.aspx

Pillemer, K., Hegeman, C., Albright, B. and Henderson, C. (1998) Building bridges between families and nursing home staff: The partners in caregiving program, *The Gerontologist*, 38(4): 499–503.

Ryan, A. and Scullion, H. (2000a) Family and staff perceptions of the role of families in nursing homes, *Journal of Advanced Nursing*, 32(3): 626–34.

Ryan, A. and Scullion, H. (2000b) Nursing home placement: An exploration of the experiences of family carers, *Journal of Advanced Nursing*, 32: 1187–95.

Sortland, O. (2020) 'Distribution of gifts and tasks', PhD thesis, University of Bergen.

Stranz, A. and Szebehely, M. (2018) Organizational trends impacting on everyday realities: The case of Swedish eldercare, in K. Christensen and D. Pilling (eds) *The Routledge Handbook of Social Care Work Around the World*, Routledge, pp 45–57.

Szebehely, M. (2017) Residential care for older people: Are there lessons to be learned from Sweden? *Journal of Canadian Studies*, 50(2): 499–507.

Utley-Smith, Q., Colon-Emeric, C., Lekan-Rutledge, D., Ammarell, N., Bailey, D., Corazzini, K., et al (2009) Staff perceptions of staff-family interactions in nursing homes, *Journal of Aging Studies*, 23: 168–77.

Ward-Griffin, C., Bol, N., Hay, K. and Dashnay, I. (2003) Relationships between families and registered nurses in long-term care facilities: A critical analysis, *Canadian Journal of Nursing Research*, 35(4): 150–74.

8

Contextual conditions and social mechanisms in rural communities and care homes

Oddrunn Sortland, Petra Ulmanen and James Struthers

In this chapter we explore contextual and social mechanisms in rural areas in Sweden, Norway and Ontario, Canada, and how they create and shape interactions between older people in care homes, their families, the staff and the volunteers. Geographical and physical conditions frame the outer context and impact service provision and how people relate to each other.

As was pointed out in Chapter 1, there are similarities and distinctions between the availability of care home beds, staff, competence and volunteers that both inform and complicate comparative analysis across jurisdictions. We draw on similar characteristics in four rural sites across jurisdictional and regional boundaries, condensing and analysing central themes that emerged in interviews and fieldnotes.

There are significant differences regarding how services are arranged and organised nationally, regionally, municipally and geographically. This affects home care provision and the level of needs required to be assigned to move into a care home (Chapter 2). As Martens (2017) argues, in Norway, region and postal code affect the availability and amount of care provision, and care is not equally distributed among older people in the country. In our experience, there are also significant differences in access across different regions in both Ontario and Sweden.

Long distances between scattered settlements make multiple daily visits from home-care services and the availability of professional care difficult (Daatland and Veenstra 2012). In sparsely populated rural municipalities, smaller and tighter groups of care workers are providing care in older people's homes. This facilitates personal relationships and continuity in care. Care workers in rural areas also report closer cooperation between different organisational units providing services to elderly. As Sortland (2020), Ulmanen (2018) and Masvie and Ytrehus (2013) argue in a Nordic rural context, personal and professional knowledge supports the flow of necessary information and reduces the social distance among groups of staff. This is also likely to be the case in Ontario.

Geographical conditions also influence relationships between older people and their offspring. It is more common for different generations of a family to live as neighbours in rural areas, but also common for family members to live further apart as younger generations move to urban areas (Hjälm, 2011; Herlofson and Daatland, 2016; Poulin, 2021). In addition, historically, urban areas have had closer proximity to a variety of medical and professional care services, which are sparser in rural areas, where people are more dependent on family, neighbours and local community (Sortland, 2020).

Shorter ([1975] 1979) describes how historically village life in the countryside impacted interactions between inhabitants. Social transparency in the local community reduced the privacy of individuals and families and created strong normative guidelines for what one could and could not do. This posed numerous threats to reputations and status, and reached into every aspect of daily life. Shorter ([1975] 1979) refers to this phenomenon as 'the tyranny of the community'. In urban areas, with high population density and more anonymity, the degree of social transparency is significantly diminished, and this affects social mechanisms and how people relate to one another in private and professional life (Sortland, 2020).

Anonymity is sparse in rural environments, and the distinction between private and public roles and spheres is fluid. This can present challenges for staff in health and care home units, who must negotiate conflicts in the local community, deal with enquiries made during their leisure time, and maintain confidentiality. However, it also has the advantage of knowledge of the older person and their family, which can lead to greater staff involvement in care work, and the creation of strong relationships between caregiver and care recipient (Masvie and Ytrehus, 2013; De Smedt and Mehus, 2017).

Lack of anonymity is challenging when older people and their families meet neighbours or acquaintances who they would rather did not have access to sensitive information (Andersen, 2011). Eika et al (2014) also describe how residents' reputations have significance for how staff treat them in the care home units. Common knowledge of people and places, however, makes it easier to find topics of conversation and establish relationships. The result of these Norwegian studies and the underlying social mechanisms described are also transferrable to Sweden and Ontario.

Theoretical framework

Building relationships and 'helping out' are important social mechanisms at work in transparent and tight communities, as we have observed in this study. This practical sense of investment and reciprocity have implications for unpaid care.

The pursuit of recognition captures many aspects of human actions, and is usually an unconscious and deeply integrated way of being. Bourdieu ([1980]

2007) operates with the concepts of economic, cultural, social and symbolic capital, where the symbolic is first and foremost linked to an individual's way of being. Prieur (2006) argues that the pursuit of symbolic capital can be used as an explanation for much of what we do in our social lives.

Being generous in the distribution of practical and symbolic gifts such as services and help provides the giver with a form of reputation and puts the recipient in a position where he or she repays with respect and a form of gratitude (Mauss, [1950] 2015). Social spaces and contexts are the bearers of collective rules of the game of both a legal and a normative nature (Bourdieu, [1980] 2007). The participants achieve a form of social prestige by complying with current norms and rules of the game. Excesses, on the other hand, entail a risk of loss of token capital and position. Contributing to the local community can both serve as an investment strategy and as a reciprocal safety net, building social and symbolic capital that is useful in both the long and the short term. This social mechanism also works in urban areas, but in other ways, and it is less pronounced.

Method and data

The method used for this study is described and discussed in Chapter 1. We compare and analyse data from fieldnotes and interviews with residents, family members, volunteers and staff working in different positions in care homes. These include managers, registered nurses (RNs), assistant nurses and personal support workers, with an emphasis on characteristics of the rural care homes rather than the urban ones.

The data are from two urban homes with 107 and 174 residents, and two rural homes with 50 and 56 beds in Norway; from an urban home with 38 residents and a rural home with 59 residents in Sweden; and from two urban homes with 450 and 256 beds, respectively, and a rural home with 112 beds in Ontario.

Together the analysed data consist of interviews with 29 residents, 46 family members, 37 members of staff and 8 volunteers, with fieldnotes providing an essential contribution to showing how people interact and relate to each other beyond what can be understood from interviews.

Geographical conditions

Families of residents often go through a struggle to get their older relative assigned a care home bed. There are differences between how this stress was experienced in the three jurisdictions and in the urban and rural sites in this study. (Differences in the experiences of family members in Ontario and Sweden are described in Chapter 2.) Family members in the urban sites more often talked about performing extensive care and advocating for their older relatives before and during the period of their being assigned a bed. A daughter of a female resident in Norway explained that this struggle lasted almost a year:

'We worked for that (getting a permanent place in a care home) for a long time, as we thought she should get a place there sooner. We applied, and were denied, and applied and were denied. In the end, I called the Patient Rights Office and asked if we didn't have a right. He confirmed that we did. I then called the municipality and said that I had talked to the Patient Rights Office and had been told that Mother was entitled to get a place, and that I hoped that they intended to do something about it, so I didn't have to involve the Patient Rights Office. Then she got a place quite fast. And at that time we were quite desperate. ... She started to forget, had a lot of pain, and used strong painkillers, and felt very much alone at home.'

The struggle in the assignment process is further complicated for family members who might feel a burden of guilt and insecurity for not being able to care for their elderly relatives and having to place them in a care home in the hands of others. Although problems related to reapplying were less often raised in interviews with families in rural sites, some families in both urban and rural sites encountered encouraging and helpful home-care staff and management during the assignment process. Especially for family members struggling to preserve their own physical and mental health, it was a relief to be supported in applying for a care home bed (Chapter 2).

If they do not have family and services in close proximity, frail older adults in rural areas may be more at risk when their health and function levels are declining and they have a need for permanent placement in a care home. Greater distances make it harder and more expensive for home care to meet their needs, which also means care home placements may happen at an earlier stage than in urban areas. This is supported by statistics from 2019 related to the Swedish urban and rural sites represented in this study. Older adults living at home in the rural municipality received 43 hours of home care per month before moving into a care home, compared to 78 hours per month in the urban municipality (NBHW, 2019). These numbers suggest that a higher level of needs is probably required to get a care home bed in the urban municipality.

Visits from family and friends

Family members, residents and staff stressed how important it was that a resident's relatives lived near their care home, because it facilitated frequent visits and intergenerational contact. As an Ontario male resident put it: "Ten-minute drive. Only a ways … I wouldn't be here without a family. I love my family." In several cases location was essential when choosing a care home. A Swedish female resident living in a care home 500 km away from her son, agreed to move into an urban home closer to him. After visiting several homes, he chose the one closest to his house, just a few minutes' walk away. He refers to it as a good and comfortable home and adds: "That is the good thing, I guess, and the proximity to us so that we can come around. I can come around maybe every second day … just to see that everything works."

Family members in rural areas commonly lived or worked some distance from the care home, which often resulted in fewer visits. The younger generation also tends to move to urban areas for study or work, making it more difficult for them to maintain relationships with the older generation. This factor was especially prominent in the Swedish sites, where families were significantly more frequent visitors to the urban home, as reflected in interviews with both staff and family members. As a care worker in a rural home said, "For their [the family's] sake and for the residents' sake, I think they come too seldom". On the other hand, as we saw from examples in the rural homes, when there is no family living close by, old friends and neighbours might visit more often.

Great distances from family might be a bigger problem in Ontario rural care homes, owing to long waiting lists and the need to accept whatever placement is available (see Chapter 2). We found residents in the rural home who were separated from their families by long distances: "I don't have family out here. I have a lot of family in the city. … Yeah, [the] distance is far enough" (Interview with male resident). Another resident, from a city an hour's drive away, ended up in the rural home "(cause) this one was the first one that had a bed come up so I was all for it. I wasn't going to wait. I wasn't going to the bottom of the level, which, you know, happens" (Interview with male resident). As Poulin (2021) points out, physical and emotional displacement from an intimate network can negatively impact older people's physical and psychological health.

Access to services, competences and staff

Location and size of care homes affect the availability of qualified staff, services, and social and cultural activities. Urban homes usually have hospitals and clinics nearby, but long distances make it difficult for rural homes to access advanced medical care. Care homes with more residents, staff, families and volunteers, as is often the case in urban locations, tend to have more diverse resources to 'play with'. That is, they have opportunities that, if explored and used, bring joy and activities into the care home.

The largest care home represented in this study, an urban home with 450 residents in Ontario, was an example of this. It has a large pool of professional skills and creative artistic talents among the staff, family members and volunteers. Together they facilitated innovative and well-attended social and cultural activities. In addition, the family council carried out effective advocacy on behalf of the residents. Larger care homes also have the space to accommodate diverse group activities and events, and may also bring in joyful elements from the outside world (see Chapter 3). Still, large is not necessarily synonymous with joyful. The potential that large homes hold must also be encouraged and managed by engaged individuals and groups who feel a sense of ownership and pride in doing so.

Location affects the composition of the workforce, and we detected a higher level of formal competence among staff in urban care homes in all three countries. Proximity to health educational institutions made it easier to recruit new employees, and access to a variety of advanced training programmes facilitated a higher degree of specialised competence among staff. Rural homes, on the other hand, faced challenges recruiting qualified staff, especially RNs. Still, they had the advantage of a lower turnover. Continuity in care settings is critical to the quality of care for residents, family and staff. There were few complaints about the formal competence of staff, however. In fact, several family members and residents at the rural sites expressed appreciation for the informal competence of staff, related to their long experience playing a key role in creating a sense of "home".

Fluidity of private and professional spheres in rural communities

In rural communities and care homes, the distinction between private and public roles and spheres is fluid. Even if they're not directly acquainted, most residents, staff, families and volunteers can relate to one another in ways related to their shared experiences outside the care home. We argue that prior knowledge of people and places *does* matter, but in different ways and degrees, which are related to the local and social context of the community and care home.

Sense of community and transparency

Historical, geographic and symbolic ties between a care home and the local community influence how, and if, people experience a feeling of ownership and engage in the inner life of the care home. This was emphasised in the municipally owned rural home in Ontario. A longstanding volunteer explained this by saying: "Well, this town is very committed to this place. Because it was – the money was raised for it locally, partly … I get the feeling that there's a sense of ownership to the home in this town." A staff fundraiser for the home's foundation stressed that the strong sense of small-town community made her job easier. "It is a place for 'neighbours taking care of neighbours'." This offered the feeling of a close-knit community in the care home, creating a strong sense of pride and ownership that generated a rich social life between visitors, staff, residents and volunteers.

The Norwegian rural home, in contrast, did not have the same relationship to the community. Although it was modern and comfortable, it had been relocated because of centralisation of services and lower-priced land, disconnecting it from the villages it had served a decade earlier. The very experienced manager argued that this had reduced the earlier intensive engagement of family members and volunteers. A lack of attachment to the home was echoed in interviews with residents and family, with most complaining about its location in "no-man's land", without any natural connection to a local community. As is argued in Chapter 9, this creates social, cultural and physical barriers for the outside community, limiting their involvement in the care home.

There are both differences and similarities between the rural sites in all three countries. They do, however, still share some of the same characteristics, which influences interactions and relationships between the different parties.

Prior knowledge as a catalyst for interaction

Prior knowledge shared between and among staff, residents, family and volunteers was a central theme in interviews conducted in the rural homes. Ontario rural residents especially, commented positively on knowing most of the staff before they moved into the home. As one replied, "Oh, I think I knew just about all of them. … They're all from [name of town]. That's an advantage of being in a small community". A manager confirmed this shared knowledge by saying, "I always joke that everybody in here is related to everybody else. Or they went to school together or they were neighbours or whatever". Another manager stated that this influenced how people related to one another: "There's definitely a lot of people looking out for one another, which I think is very important."

This prior knowledge also facilitated relationships between family members and friends. A daughter noted that since her father had been relocated to the home, "I've reconnected with three friends that I hadn't seen for years. And even one who doesn't live here any more. Their parents ended up here". Sharing both a common history and a role as a visitor in a care home offered her the opportunity to resume friendships and a feeling of togetherness in a situation that might be difficult to handle. As Mauss ([1950] 2015) argues, social and emotional support creates and shapes binding relationships in which friends can expect to support each other in caring for their elders. This mechanism works best when people know who the other is, which makes it possible to adjust their efforts of 'helping out' and predict what the response might be.

Some residents also had the advantage of prior friendships and of meeting old acquaintances. A female resident in an Ontario rural home noted that her roommate was a friend she'd known previously: "She's nice. I knew her years before. So, when we found out we're gonna be roomies, we went together happily, right?" Poor physical health, impaired hearing and reduced cognitive function can make it hard to establish relationships with other residents, but prior knowledge is a catalyst for reconnection, conversation and a feeling of togetherness with others in a similar situation. As a male Norwegian rural resident commented, "Most of those who come here know someone who is here. So there is a good atmosphere around the dining table".

Up- and downsides of shared knowledge

Most staff considered shared knowledge to be a positive thing, which strengthened trust, facilitated cooperation with family, and enabled adjustments to care. However, there were also downsides, as explained by a manager in the Ontario rural home:

'It makes some of the things we do much more difficult because when we have issues or incidents, often it's a person who's meaningful to the staff or physicians, so a death or a trauma or whatever usually touches people in the organisation personally, which we need to be respectful of, you know … it leads to a level of care and attention that … you'll know you find in small towns.'

The social transparency was somewhat lower in the Norwegian rural home, but still prominent. As an RN said:

'When you meet a new resident or family [member], they ask, "What is your name? … OK, so you are from that family?" And then I say, "No, not that family, the other". "OK, then I know who you are" or "Then I know where you belong". This is standard procedure. You have to tell if you come from this or that family. And they might say, "Yes, I knew your grandmother" or "I am the cousin of your grandfather".'

An assistant nurse said: "There are some … I don't know *them*, but they know *me*, cause they know my parents. And they are very positive, and I get a bit [of goodwill] for free." The fact that her parents had a good reputation in the local community positively affected how she was perceived by residents and family members. On the other hand, there was a downside to this, as reflected in an interview with another assistant nurse: "Not everyone thinks it is OK to expose what family you belong to. We ought to be seen as *health care workers*, and not something else. Maybe you are judged even before getting a chance to show who you are."

Some staff found it difficult to draw the line between their private and professional positions. In the rural home, an RN who formerly had a prominent position in the municipality's health-care system complained about enquiries from people at the grocery shop or phone calls to her house, making her feel she was constantly at work. She underscored however, that knowledge of a resident's family made it easier to understand family dynamics: "In small communities we might know about problems in a family, and that there is a history that explains why they are not there [for the resident] as we would expect, so that's an advantage that has been useful for me several times." Another RN confirmed this: "We sometimes wonder, "Why doesn't this nice man get any visits? But then you get to know ... this is a small place and then you hear the story of what a terrible father he has been, and all pieces fall into place."

The social transparency not only affected how care recipients were perceived by staff, but also how staff performed their daily work and maintained relations with residents and family members. When asked what it was like working and living in the same rural community, a Norwegian RN said: "I believe we are concerned about being well regarded as good health workers. 'Cause here ... it is not a big place, and we are all concerned about doing a good job and getting a good reputation." Another RN agreed that local transparency might impact their work: "Some [staff] might push themselves too hard, depending on who that person is, not to get a bad reputation. But I think most are relaxed about it as long as they feel they are doing it [their job] right."

In short, working and living in the same local community had its up- and downsides. Although none of the residents or families interviewed expressed concerns about receiving help from staff they already knew, it is likely there are some examples. This was reflected in an interview with a Swedish assistant nurse who said that she would like to live in the home where she worked *if* it were located somewhere else: "It's a good care home." She stressed that it *had* to be a good home, as negative experiences and stories spread rapidly in a transparent local environment. She did not want to live in a care home close to where she was born and raised, and said:

'I want to be more anonymous. I would not like, for instance, if I got a stroke, I don't want people to talk in the grocery shop like "I visited my wife in the care home yesterday and then I saw [her name] and she looked terrible". I think you can be too exposed in a small place like this. ... Everybody knows each other. I have a friend whose father got dementia and they put him in a care home in another village just because of that. ... I mean, we go out for walks with the residents and they are so visible to everyone, like "there he is, he who used to be the bus driver for 50 years and now, see what he looks like". It's about dignity.'

Nevertheless, the mechanisms of social control in a small local community contributed to feelings of trust, as residents and family members personally knew the families of some of the staff. If something went wrong, the consequences would likely be noticeable at a personal and social level for the staff, and a possible threat to their symbolic capital in their private sphere.

Unpaid work of family and staff

As highlighted in Chapter 1, staffing levels differ greatly between Norway and Sweden on the one hand, and Ontario on the other. Levels of staffing influence the dependence on voluntary and unpaid work, which is sometimes essential for meeting residents' physical, psychological and social needs. Although families and volunteers in Ontario might need to perform extended care work, this is rare in a Norwegian and Swedish context, where families visit, monitor the care, accompany relatives to medical appointments, and make sure residents have what they need in terms of clothing and shoes. Some contribute socially to the wards, not solely by interacting with 'their' residents, but by talking to other residents too, by making conversation, laughing and creating a friendly atmosphere. Others occasionally do some cleaning or assist their relative with eating, and sometimes help other residents, if they find it meaningful and rewarding. But families in Norwegian and Swedish care homes are seen as guests, and not as unpaid workers.

More unpaid work by staff in rural areas?

We detected unpaid work in both urban and rural contexts across national borders, and as expected, to a much higher degree from families, volunteers and staff in the three Ontario sites in this study. Still, there seems to be a higher level of unpaid work among staff in the rural homes, at least in Norway and Ontario. Armstrong's (2013) report shows that women tend to do more unpaid work than men, and this is particularly true of women with low incomes. In our study, staff in the rural care homes had fewer formal qualifications. In Norway, especially, assistant nurses often worked part time involuntarily, even competing to do extra shifts to get a decent income. Extending themselves and doing unpaid work is one of several ways to build social and symbolic capital that might be useful both in terms of employment and in other social settings.

A characteristic of the rural sites was that most staff, residents, family members and volunteers were born and raised in the local community.

Feelings of ownership, prior knowledge and personal relationships helped to motivate unpaid work on the part of staff and volunteers. A finding supporting this argument was that staff with fewer social connections to the local community, because they had moved to the area as adults, expressed a more sharply differentiated sense of professional status and a resistance to unpaid work. We argue that familiarity, community and blurred and flexible boundaries between private and professional positions and spheres in rural care homes and communities encourage or force families and staff to invest time and energy in unpaid work.

Rural homes offer both a safety net and surveillance

Although national, regional, municipal and local contexts provide different frameworks and opportunities, social mechanisms that structure human practices are similar, affecting people's social practices and ways of living and relating. People living in areas with low population density have historically been dependent on help from the local community and on solidarity with each other, because of limited access to 'professional' help in the event of illness and distress. In rural areas, there is more physical distance between people with similar interests and orientation, and the importance of finding fellowship with those who live in the immediate areas is greater.

Material or cultural capital can create distance between people, while symbolic capital that might be gained through courtesy, helpfulness or willingness to volunteer acts as a lubrication of the social machinery across social spheres and segments. Helping others is one of several ways of gaining symbolic capital, especially when other forms of capital are sparse or have less significance in social settings.

When residents, families and staff have close relationships, as is often the case in tight or rural communities, there is more at stake, which means that they increase their efforts and commitment. In social interactions in tight communities and rural areas, an unconscious understanding of the social transparency in relationships with others seemed to be physically and cognitively embedded. This works both as a form of safety net and social surveillance.

Looking after each other and offering help is a social practice that provides symbolic capital in terms of a beneficial reputation and social capital in the local community. As Sortland (2020) argues, this may be an unconscious strategy aimed at accumulating symbolic capital, which is recognised as a viable currency in all social sectors. Participating in various forms of unpaid work in nursing homes can act as a catalyst for symbolic capital in rural areas and tight communities, where social transparency is greater than in a more anonymised urban context. These are not conscious calculations of individuals but lie primarily as learned, embodied, physical and cognitive patterns of action.

If staff behave in a way for which there is little social acceptance, there is a real possibility that this will become known in the local community, and backfire in the form of a bad reputation and reduced symbolic capital. It can therefore be argued that the relationship between providers and recipients of services is to some extent structured by whether it occurs in an urban or rural context.

Policy implications

As Poulin argues, it is essential to 'recognize that large catchment areas, displacement and universal models of care foster inequitable services in rural areas' (Poulin 2021, p 4). This disparity applies to residents living in the care homes examined in all three jurisdictions reviewed in this chapter. Less accessible home-care options make nursing home care a more urgent priority for rural families, yet even when available, their care home beds are located farther away from advanced medical care than what is on offer to their urban counterparts.

Physical distances separating residents from their friends and loved ones in rural settings may also be much greater than in urban contexts. Smaller rural care homes also have fewer paid and unpaid resources for providing high-quality social activities to their residents than homes in urban areas. In addition, rural homes have less access to higher levels of staff competence and training. In rural homes in Ontario, there also appears to be a much greater dependence on the unpaid care work performed by family members, staff and volunteers. Funding and governance models which do not take account of these fundamental disparities will continue to ensure a significantly lower quality of life for care home residents living in rural contexts.

References

Andersen, T.H. (2011) Det er slik livet er: Perspektiver fra et forskningsprosjekt om menn som primære omsorgspersoner for partner/ektefelle med betydelig omsorgsbehov [That's how life is: Perspectives from a research project of men as primary caregivers for partners/spouses with extended care needs], Research Report, Center for Care Research. Available from: http://hdl.handle.net/11250/144328

Armstrong, P. (2013) Unpaid Health Care: An Indicator for Equity, Pan American Health Organization.

Bourdieu, P. ([1980] 2007) Den praktiske sans [The practical sense], trans Peer F. Bundgård, Hans Reitzelts Forlag.

Daatland, S.O. and Veenstra, M. (2012) Lokale variasjoner i eldreomsorgen, in S.O. Daatland and M. Veenstra (eds) Bærekraftig omsorg: Familien, velferdsstaten og aldringen av befolkningen [Sustainable care: The family, the welfare state and the aging society], Report 2/12, NOVA–Norwegian Social Research Institute, pp 79–108.

De Smedt, S.E. and Mehus, G. (2017) Sykepleieforskning i rurale områder i Norge: en scoping review [Local variations in care for elderly nursing research in rural areas in Norway: A scoping review], *Nordisk tidsskrift for helseforskning*, 13(2), https://doi.org/10.7557/14.4238

Eika, M., Espnes, G.A., and Hvalvik, S. (2014) Nursing staff's actions during older residents' transition into long-term care facility in a nursing home in rural Norway, *International Journal of Qualitative Studies on Health and Well-Being*, 9(1): 1–12, https://doi.org/10.3402/qhw.v9.24105

Herlofson, K. and Daatland, S.O. (2016) *Forskning om familiegenerasjoner. En kunnskapsstatus* [Research on family generations: A knowledge status], Research Report 2/2016, NOVA–Norwegian Social Research Institute.

Hjälm, A. (2011) 'A family landscape: On the geographical distances between elderly parents and adult children in Sweden', PhD thesis, Umeå University, Sweden.

Martens, C.T. (2017) 'Allocating responsibilities: Norwegian elder care between national ambitions and local autonomy', PhD thesis, University of Oslo.

Masvie, T.B. and Ytrehus, S. (2013) Psykisk helsearbeideres erfaringer med å jobbe i små kommuner i Nordland [Mental health workers experience on working on small municipalities in Northern Norway], *Nordisk tidsskrift for helseforskning*, 9(1): 19–34.

Mauss, M. ([1950] 2015) *Gaven: Utvekslingers form og årsak i arkaiske samfunn* [The gift: Forms and functions of exchange in archaic societies], trans Thomas Hylland Eriksen, Cappelens akademisk forlag.

National Board of Health and Welfare (NBHW, Sweden) (2019) *Enhetsundersökningen om äldreomsorg och kommunal hälso- och sjukvård* [The unit survey on elderly care and municipal health care], Article 2019–10–6419, Socialstyrelsen.

Poulin, L. (2021) *A Plan of Action: 11 Recommendations to Enhance Long-term Care Provision in Canada: Insights from a Project on the Transitional Care of Rural Older Adults*, Trent Centre for Aging & Society.

Prieur, A. (2006) En teori om praksis [A theory of practice], in A. Prieur and C. Sestoft (eds) *Pierre Bourdieu*, Hanz Reitzels Forlag, pp 23–71.

Shorter, E. ([1975] 1979) *Kernefamiliens historie* [The making of the modern family] (trans Lars Stubbe Teglbjærg), Nyt Nordisk Forlag.

Sortland, O. (2020) 'Fordeling av gaver og oppgaver: En praxeologisk studie av hjelpe- og utvekslingspraksiser mellom eldre med hjelpebehov, familien og ansatte i kommunal eldreomsorg' [Distribution of gifts and tasks: A praxeological study of exchange practices between elderly people in need of help, the family and employees in municipal elderly care], PhD thesis, University of Bergen.

Ulmanen, P. (2018) Anhörigomsorg i stad och land [Family care in cities and countryside], in H. Jönson and M. Szebehely (eds) *Äldreomsorger i Sverige: lokala variationer och generella trender*, Gleerups Utbildning AB, pp 201–16.

9

Bringing the outside in and the inside out: the role of institutional boundaries in nursing homes

Frode F. Jacobsen and Gudmund Ågotnes

This chapter offers an analysis based on ethnographic research in six Norwegian nursing homes with different degrees and forms of integration into local communities, with community understood as the local neighbourhood, a village or a city. In addition to the Norwegian research undertaken in the five years before the pandemic, the analysis is informed by fieldwork carried out in nursing homes in Canada, the UK, the US and Sweden, adding an international, comparative dimension to our analysis.

Exploring the boundaries between the outside and inside of care homes, we show the importance of the permeability of these boundaries not only to residents, families and staff, but also to the wider community. These boundaries are particularly relevant to those crossing them when moving into the care home, and to the family members and significant others accompanying them (see Chapter 2). More broadly, exploring these boundaries entails investigating the presence and significance of the outside community in the nursing homes, and of the nursing homes in the outside community. With this as a starting point, we ask if, how and to what degree nursing homes can constitute forms of 'community' themselves, influencing and being influenced by the wider community. We argue that the nature of the boundaries has consequences for forms of unpaid work in nursing homes, both in terms of what this work entails and where it is performed.

We focus on the cultural, social and physical dimensions of the boundaries of the six institutions. As Chapter 1 puts it, the people who live in nursing homes represent some of the most vulnerable in our society, providing a way to assess the economic, political, cultural and social conditions of the larger society, as well as its values. We argue that a high level of protective measures in nursing homes, resulting in solidifying their boundaries to make them less permeable, will increase vulnerability among residents. Even the nicest natural surroundings cannot compensate for social isolation and for the absence of the non-professional care of families and friends.

A case from Western Norway

The following account raises an important question: What relationship should nursing homes have with the communities surrounding them?

> Several residents of the small Norwegian city have expressed their concerns on social media about a new street constructed outside the nursing home, stressing that the older residents deserve peace and quiet instead of noise from workers and construction site engines. The older residents living there disagree. One male resident states that "Nowadays I experience some variation in the view [from my window]. People ask me if I experience long days here. I answer that there is so much to observe [connected to the construction activities]". A woman says that she would not move to a less central and more quiet beauty spot if she got the choice. Another woman supports her, stating that "It is important to have a view of things moving and changing. I like to watch children merrily walking and partly jumping on their way to school".
>
> In another Norwegian small city, a panoramic view of the mountains and the fjord was supposed to be "the icing on the cake" of a newly constructed nursing home. However, merely two of the new residents have chosen a room with the panoramic view. The rest of them wanted a room on the rear side of the building, which looked out towards the main road, a shopping mall, the primary school and the sports grounds. (NRK, 2022, trans. Jacobsen)

In the context of COVID and conflicting concerns about infection spread and resident isolation, we analyse how nursing homes relate to their close social and physical environments, highlighting the significance for residents, staff, family members and the wider community. The relationship between the institution and the world beyond is under-studied, with most research maintaining its gaze within the walls of the nursing home. We argue that these relationships are decisive for whether residents experience a meaningful life, and should be considered in the analysis of unpaid work in nursing homes.

In this chapter, questions of unpaid work are approached somewhat differently than in other chapters. First, we describe the presence of unpaid work in nursing homes by addressing issues of access to and mobility within nursing homes, as opposed to the types and impacts of unpaid work. Second, our starting point is that the forms of unpaid work, particularly work that brings 'the outside in' and situations where 'the inside is taken out', may sometimes be beneficial and complementary to the paid work inside nursing homes. Unpaid work may enhance social activities, strengthen connections to the community outside of the walls of the nursing home, and in general, create a meaningful social life for the residents. Hence, we focus on forms of unpaid work that need not be exploitative by nature and which can be facilitated what we label the 'unbracketing' of nursing homes, namely making the boundaries more permeable to a flow of persons, activities and goods, and to non-professional love and care, to wider social relationships, adding to as opposed to replacing the important and wide-ranging professional care work. Although the nursing home examples introduced in the chapter represent Norwegian cases, we hold this insight to be valid beyond the Norwegian jurisdiction.

In the past, Norwegian nursing homes were often built in peaceful and quiet surroundings, with a view of a beautiful landscape, and many of those still exist today. As with the tuberculosis sanatoria and early psychiatric hospitals, the dominant idea among professionals and society in general was that peace and quiet would do residents good. Nursing homes were conceived as institutions offering serenity, but also as institutions keeping the residents from the outside: as a kind of container of frail people. The idea of the nursing home was akin to Goffman's notion of a 'total institution' (Goffman, 1961), or to the notion of a sort of 'bracket' or an 'other space' in ordinary society (Foucault and Miskowiec, 1986).

Although the stress on peace and quiet for frail older adults is less pronounced now, the location of newer institutions still implies a degree of isolation from society – from organised public events, or spontaneous activities such as people gathering in a park when the weather is nice. And while investment in staff and buildings has been relatively high in the Norwegian nursing home sector (Hauge and Heggen, 2008; Harrington et al, 2012; Jacobsen, 2021), there has been less attention directed at the social and physical environments of the nursing homes. This chapter explores the relationship of nursing homes to their social and physical surroundings through case studies from ethnographic fieldwork in six Norwegian nursing homes during the period 2014–19. To set the context, we provide a brief background of the Norwegian nursing home sector.

Norwegian nursing homes

Norway has a tradition of prioritising residential care for older adults. Although the numbers are declining, around 12 per cent of the Norwegian population over 80 lives in nursing homes (Statistics Norway, 2021) and in 2019, approximately 45 per cent of all deaths among people over 60 occurred in an nursing home (Statistics Norway, 2020). Norwegian nursing homes are regulated by health-care legislation and are considered health institutions (Jacobsen, 2015). Together, nursing homes and the small but growing supportive housing sector can be characterised as a long-term residential care system of 'two regimes', where supportive housing is frequently associated with 24/7 health and care services, communal meals and common rooms (Daatland et al, 2015).

In the Nordic countries, care for older people is the responsibility of local authorities (Andersson, 2011; Stig et al, 2013). Still, the nursing home sector is characterised by greater uniformity than in other parts of Europe and in the US (Graverholt et al, 2013), for example, in how nursing homes are equipped, staffed and operated. While home-based care is increasingly prioritised, in Norway, nursing homes play a more significant role in the care of the frailest older people than in most other European countries (OECD, 2022).

The investment in nursing home buildings has been high in Norway since 2000, after a White Paper declared that all shared resident rooms must be transformed into single rooms (Ministry of Health and Social Affairs, 1996–97). The official goal was precisely formulated as at least 90 per cent single occupancy by 2005 (Ministry of Social Affairs, 2001–02), with shared bathrooms converted into single bathrooms. By 2020, this was the case with 90.4 per cent of the rooms (Statistics Norway, 2021). This nationwide rebuilding included transforming larger wards into smaller ones of 4 to 12 residents, a development often linked to the objective of creating so-called dementia-friendly environments (Høyland et al, 2015). In line with all the Nordic countries, this rebuilding is intended to promote the home-like environments seen as the ideal for frail older adults (Andersson, 2011). The balance between the ideal of a home-like environment and a professional health institution, the latter required by law, is a matter for continual debate in Norway (Hauge, 2004; Jacobsen, 2021).

Relations with the wider community: physical and social surroundings

In Norway, there is an increasing awareness of the importance of the immediate surroundings to nursing homes (Høyland et al, 2018). This has, for instance, materialised in the form of sensory gardens, a type of green environment accessible to people with disabilities and stimulating for persons with dementia and other frail older people. There is also a growing public awareness of the aesthetic and social advantages of the built and natural environments of nursing homes, including their access to shopping malls, cultural centres, restaurants and parks (Høyland et al, 2018; Jacobsen and Sundsbø, 2020).

This growing awareness seems to have had limited real-life consequences for the location of new nursing homes. A study of the more than 30 nursing homes in Bergen, the second-largest Norwegian city, indicate that newer institutions are less accessible to cafés, restaurants, schools, kindergartens, parks, playgrounds, libraries, sports arenas, cinemas and shopping malls.

Decreased accessibility is a result both of geographical distance and of physical and psychological barriers such as traffic-congested roads, walls, stairways and camera-surveilled entries (Jacobsen, 2014, p 270).

The co-location of nursing homes with various public services and semi-public facilities like libraries, supportive housing, kindergartens, gyms, swimming pools, supermarkets and museums appears in a few rare cases. However, recent nursing home construction seems to locate them where the cost of land is relatively low. In some extreme cases they are built on manufacturing sites or even industrial wasteland, where moving outside the nursing home facility involves potential health hazards (Jacobsen, 2013).

The nursing home cases

The nursing home cases presented here are not representative of all Norwegian institutions. One reason is that some of them have been selected for an international study of promising practices (https://reltc.apps01.yorku. ca), and singled out on the basis of features identified as promising in research literature or by local informants. One such feature was integration of the institution into the local social and physical environment. The examples discussed still serve to illustrate how specific dimensions of nursing homes may facilitate or hinder relationships with the community, and, in general, their integration into Norwegian society.

The rebuilt nursing home

Frode Jacobsen has been carrying out fieldwork at one nursing home since 1988. This includes a renovation in 2003. The nursing home is typical of Norwegian nursing homes in size, with around 60 residents. It used to have two large units on different floors, each with 29 residents. The resident rooms, several of them double occupancies, were situated along two longer, hospital-like white corridors, one perpendicular to the other, with the nurses' station in the intersection between the two, and two large windows facing both corridors. After the renovation, three new wards of eight to ten residents were constructed out of each old ward.

Single occupancy and a change in the ward's physical structure influenced staff relationships with residents. The private rooms meant that the privacy of residents was more respected and the staff supported the dignity of the residents to a greater extent than before, for example, by avoiding so-called elderspeak, that is, speaking to older people as if they were children.

The physical division into smaller units has nearly tripled the space in the common areas. In theory, this could have contributed to more contact between the institution and the surrounding community by allowing for more meeting space between visitors and residents. In practice, however, this did not occur. Although the management emphasised in interviews a policy encouraging contact with relatives, volunteers, and people from outside in general, people other than staff and residents were rarely observed in the living rooms after the physical changes. An administration notice posted on each ward's entrance door explicitly encouraged relatives and other visitors to go straight to the room of the resident they intended to visit and to avoid the common areas, so as to 'not disturb or be disturbed by other people present in the common areas'.

This measure reinforced the home's isolation from its social surroundings. The home is located in a quiet suburb without many public venues. It is attached to a graveyard on one side and the back of a now-disused school on the other. This example illustrates how physical surroundings and administrative routines combined can facilitate or hinder social interaction with the wider society. These factors contribute to the institution appearing as a separate and sequestered place in the local community. In turn, this could explain some of the everyday social life in this nursing home, like the unusual sound level in several wards. A television set dominates the living room, with a level of sound so high that both residents and staff almost have to shout in order to communicate. In contrast, meals are frequently consumed in close to total silence, a situation that does not fit well with Norwegian cultural expectations of meals in people's own homes, where the normal situation would be that people chat amiably during a meal (Jacobsen, 2015).

Boundaries between inside and outside

Our second case is from a similarly sized nursing home (around 60 residents), built several decades later, in accordance with the new criteria. Almost all rooms are single occupancy with bathrooms, and the home is divided into smaller units with long corridors and a large common area in each. This home is located on the outskirts of a sparsely populated area and is difficult to get to without the use of a car although there is a bus connection. In other words, it is not directly connected to a community. A resident cannot walk from the nursing home to a nearby neighbourhood. Perhaps because of this, the area surrounding the nursing home was given particular attention during construction, and includes an elaborate sensory garden. The garden was intended as a physical and aesthetic centrepiece and a gathering point for residents and families, somewhere to walk when receiving visitors or with staff members, and aimed to offer attractive views from the residents' rooms or the common areas. However, the garden was neglected, and after a few years, all that remained were dead shrubs and plants. One of the staff members explained that the maintenance of the garden had fallen under a different municipal division than the one overseeing nursing home care, leading to a situation where nobody was responsible, or at least nobody knew who was responsible.

The case illustrates how the boundaries of nursing homes, seemingly both trivial and distinct, can take different forms, where the physical walls signify one type of boundary, and the physical property, including the immediate area outside the walls, another.

Bringing the inside out

At the same nursing home, the presence of 'the outside' was limited, except for family members visiting residents. One remarkable exception is worthy of mention, however. On the 17 May national holiday, the nearest kindergarten came visiting. In typical national holiday tradition, the small children walked in a parade, in their best clothes, waving flags, while singing and wishing those they passed a joyful celebration. They walked through each ward, where almost all of the residents were lined up, waving back at them. A nurse at the care home was moved by the scene, crying silently as the children walked by.

This example illustrates how the ways in which the outside is brought into the nursing home can have a major impact on residents and staff. At other homes, 'the outside' is almost an integral part of the care home's internal life. A larger nursing home facilitates community interaction. Located in the middle of a residential area, near a busy intersection, it is easily accessible both by car and public transportation, and within walking distance of shops and several neighbourhoods. More importantly, the nursing home functions as a form of community centre for the local area. The large and open entrance area allows visitors space and opportunities for participating in various activities, including visiting the cafeteria, which contains a large dining area and serves low-cost meals, or spending time in a public space with the home's residents. A local group of accordion players practise at the nursing home and now and then give a performance for residents, relatives and other visitors from the community. The nursing home is part of a large non-profit organisation, which makes the nursing home a benefit to the wider local community and vice versa by inviting music groups and other local activities in the neighbourhood to practice and perform on the nursing home premises.

Bringing the outside in

Another, older nursing home is similarly located in the middle of a large residential area, with excellent access (by car, by public transportation and on foot) to local amenities and the surrounding residential area. However, aside from individual visitors, the outside community played only a small part in the nursing home's everyday life. This can, in part, be attributed to the home's physical features: it is an old building originally built as an apartment complex and later converted into an nursing home. It does not have a large and accessible common room. Being a publicly operated institution, it did not have the advantage of volunteers either. Moreover, the interior was ill-suited for moving around, especially for frail older people, owing to the narrow hallways and just one lift. Consequently, the residents tended to be secluded within the confines of their ward. However, during the summer, the staff put in considerable efforts to alleviate this situation and take the residents outside. Every day, and despite great physical barriers and time constraints, they would bring many of the residents to the area just outside the entrance, which was furnished with benches and small tables where they could sit together and take in the life of the neighbourhood. Most would simply sit there and converse, drinking lemonade, while others would join staff members for short walks or be assisted with their wheelchairs by staff members.

Where outside is inside and the inside is embedded in the outside

A nursing home in a rural community along the western coast of Norway is located at the vibrant centre of the community. The nursing home is in the same building as the cultural centre, and they share the same main entrance. The cultural centre contains, among other facilities, a library, a swimming pool, a sports hall, a gym, a concert hall, a cinema, a so-called culture café, and a sizable lobby that features historical and arts exhibitions.

This atypical collaboration between local government agencies came about after a spontaneous meeting between the Chief Medical Officer and the municipality's Head of Culture. As a result, nursing home residents can walk to the sports hall and watch their grandchildren play football or other games, and grandchildren can visit their grandparents in the nursing home after visiting the local cinema. Residents' children can drop by and say hello after visiting an adjacent shopping mall, which contains, in addition to various shops, restaurants and businesses, a doctor's office, a dental clinic and a physiotherapy clinic. The local church is close by as well.

Nursing home residents were often observed moving between different locations inside the joint nursing home and cultural centre building, often with walking frames and wheelchairs. Even more frequently, residents were spotted engaged in less demanding activities, like sitting with a panoramic view of kids and families swimming in the pool one level below, or observing people passing by on their way to shop or visit a clinic.

The nursing home is part of a continuum of care arrangement that includes ordinary housing, supportive housing and the headquarters of the home-based care services. This means that older people are able to stay at or near this municipal centre as their health and level of functioning changes.

Nursing homes in the community and wider society

As Andersson (2011) points out, the characteristics of institutions' boundaries – understood as *physical, social* and *cultural* – determine the qualities of their inner life. The more that visible and invisible walls separate the inside from the outside, the more the interior of nursing homes develops into an 'other space' in the Foucauldian sense (Foucault and Miskowiec, 1986); that is, a space separated from ordinary society. While *time* has become increasingly secularised in the sense of becoming dominantly homogeneous and linear time, secularisation of *space* has at most been partial, allowing for a heterogeneity of spaces (Foucault and Miskowiec, 1986). Places like prisons, holy sites, museums, royal properties, cemeteries, mental hospitals and institutions for older people are extraordinary in the sense of standing out from more profane spaces, by having an element of sacredness (in the sense of being set apart from the mundane and ordinary society), either positively or negatively. Such places can be described as sharing particular positive or negative characteristics, as 'there is a light, ethereal, transparent space, or again a dark, rough, encumbered space; a space from above, of summits, or on the contrary a space from below, of mud' (Foucault and Miskowiec 1986, p 23).

Following Foucault's typology of heterotopia, an institution for older people may both be regarded as a (life) crisis heterotopia, related to human life stages like adolescence and old age, and as a deviation heterotopia, 'since, in our society where leisure is the rule, idleness is a sort of deviation' (Foucault and Miskowiec, 1986, p 25). Nursing homes may be viewed as exceptional places, possibly more in a negative than positive sense, and as 'brackets' in relation to what is perceived as ordinary community or society.

The permeability of the nursing homes' physical, cultural and social boundaries relates to the degree of 'bracketisation' in the institutions. Accessibility of the inner spaces to family, volunteers, neighbours and others (such as children from schools and kindergartens) makes the inner social life of nursing homes more transparent, and hence open to judgment from and interference by the local community. Being open to people from outside, even if far from continuously, can have a 'normalising' or even civilising effect, and can stand as an example of how (unpaid) efforts or work from 'the outside' is of benefit to staff and residents alike.

Opportunities for residents to access the neighbourhood and surrounding areas affect their outlook on life and their experience of the nursing home as a home. This is because appreciating the intimacy of a home strongly relates to one's ability to access the opposite: public places (Lund, 2003). This ability can also allow more self-care. The cases above illustrate that physical and social enablers – and any barriers to them – play an important role. A routine tour of the neighbourhood is a social enabler. Posted notes on entrance doors advising visitors not to enter common areas by contrast exemplify a social barrier.

Physical barriers and enablers may, in some cases, primarily have a visual quality. Contrary to media concerns over a noisy playground or construction site, being able to watch children playing or construction workers work can make life inside the nursing home more meaningful and bearable for residents. And the cumulative effect of so-called passive, minor activities may play a larger role than that of organised events with activities which are easier for visitors to notice, like bingo or music events (Gubrium, 1975).

In the larger picture, Norwegian nursing homes appear to be secluded from the wider society – now as before – albeit in part for different reasons than in the past. To a large extent, they still offer few opportunities for residents to experience the pulsating social life outside the facility, and for people in the wider society to access and have a feel for what is happening inside the walls of the nursing homes. Although there are some notable exceptions, like the examples given of co-location, the nursing homes appear to be an example of Goffman's 'total institutions' (Goffman, 1961). For Goffman, lack of communication between the inside and outside of an institution contributes to standardised routines over which 'inmates' lack influence and control. It also fosters the breakdown of barriers between areas of everyday life normally kept separate in Western societies, like between where one eats and sleeps, works and enjoys leisure activities (Goffman, 1961). In a seminal doctoral thesis, Swedish architect and social scientist Jonas Andersson demonstrated how the degree of permeability of an nursing home's boundaries is a salient indicator of the quality of the social life inside it (Andersson, 2011). His study aligns well with Goffman's insights.

Although in the latest three decades there has been an important political movement in Norway stressing the need for opening up the previously isolated health institutions, the extent to which this has taken place is questionable. Rather, it can be argued that the majority of nursing homes are isolated from public life and from the wider society.

In fact, the accessibility of culturally important public and semi-public areas to nursing homes may have decreased. Even though investment in outdoor spaces in the form of gardens has been significant, the gardens are frequently enclosed inside buildings, tall hedges or fences and are often not maintained. At the same time as areas outside the nursing homes have not become more accessible to residents, there are also barriers against the outside world entering the nursing home. While some nursing homes actively market their dining hall as a neighbourhood cafeteria where everyone is welcome, this is still the exception rather than the rule. The small entrance areas surveilled by video cameras do not encourage volunteers and other visitors to enter the facility, but instead maintain the nursing home as a heterotopia, bracketing it off from the wider society. Posters/signs asking family and other visitors to avoid common areas and go straight to the resident's private room are a social barrier as solid and effective as a concrete wall between the outside and inside of the facility.

The social and physical environments of Norwegian nursing homes seem to support an institutional logic that undermines both the professed aim of a good last home for frail older adults, and the often heroic day-to-day struggle of the staff to create a home-like experience for residents. Such a logic undermines the ways in which (unpaid) work from 'outsiders', that is, volunteers or family members, positively contributes to the nursing homes. The position of nursing homes in society and their often-marginal geographical location seem to mirror dominating ideological trends that see chronically ill and frail older adults as outside the main focus of health policy discourse. Nursing homes today may still to some extent be considered 'containers' for the people they are housing, even though they may appear aesthetically more successful than their predecessors.

There are cultural barriers in addition to the physical and social barriers. While policy papers are significant in establishing and maintaining cultural expectations of old age and of what living in a care home is like, the role of the mass media is likely even more important. How politicians, decision-makers and journalists portray nursing homes prevents them from being viewed as a positive option for a last home or as a place to be feared and avoided.

Such barriers are also important for the extent to which volunteers, relatives, friends and people from the local community are motivated to visit and contribute to the nursing homes.

Removing the brackets from around nursing homes

Even though Norwegian nursing homes do not seem unpopular as a potential place for living the last years of one's life, and even though older people may choose or even fight to move into a nursing home in case of pronounced frailty (Munkejord et al, 2018), the cultural influences of politics and the mass media seem to pull in the opposite direction.

Moving away from nursing homes has been a trend in all the Nordic countries for several decades (Rostgaard et al, 2022). The Norwegian government has been actively promoting aging at home (Daatland, 2014). This implies directing health and care resources for older people primarily towards home-based care services, both for people living in their own homes and for those in supportive housing. Norwegian policies of aging in place appear to exemplify a romantic cultural imaginary of home as good and of the existence of untapped local resources with regard to family, neighbourhood, volunteers and companies (Löfquist et al, 2013; Meagher and Szebehely, 2013; Munkejord et al, 2018; Dalmer, 2019).

Nursing homes are, in a way, a place where one is not supposed to be, and whose mere existence testifies to a health policy failure. Still, their position appears much stronger in Norway than in the other Nordic countries (Rostgaard et al, 2022). There are few signs that nursing homes are losing their importance within society or as part of the health-care system. As in earlier times, they are still 'another space' in the Foucauldian sense (Foucault and Miskowiec, 1986).

This paradoxical situation holds some promise. Nursing homes will remain an important part of Norwegian care services for many years to come. The willingness to maintain a relatively high number of nursing home beds compared to other countries, and to invest substantial funds in improving nursing home buildings and securing a relatively high level of staff coverage and competence, indicates that aging in place is not the only ideology. Increased investment in social and physical accessibility and in integration of nursing homes into their local communities, and hence their 'unbracketing', may not be a far-fetched vision. Besides drawing attention to the many non-employees contributing to nursing homes, the still ongoing COVID-19 pandemic has highlighted worldwide the destructiveness of social isolation and the need to improve communication and social transactions between institutions and the wider society (Jacobsen et al, 2021). COVID-19 has made clear the urgent necessity of opening up, unbracketing nursing homes, in Norway and elsewhere. Unbracketing furthermore implies opening up for wider social relationships and for beneficial forms of unpaid work from families and friends. However, and in alignment with other chapters in this volume, this is a benefit that should add to, as opposed to replacing, professionalised care work.

References

Andersson, J. (2011) 'Architecture and ageing: On the interaction between frail older people and the built environment', PhD thesis, KTH Royal Institute of Technology.

Daatland, S.O. (ed) (2014) *Boliggjøring av eldreomsorgen?* [Towards a housing-oriented model in older people's care?], Report 16/2014, NOVA.

Daatland, S.O., Høyland, K. and Otnes, B. (2015) Scandinavian contrasts and Norwegian variations in special housing for older people, *Journal of Housing For the Elderly*, 29(1–2): 180–96, doi: 10.1080/02763893.2015.989778

Dalmer, N.K. (2019) A logic of choice: Problematizing the documentary reality of Canadian aging in place policies, *Journal of Aging Studies*, 48: 40–9, https://doi.org/10.1016/j.jaging.2019.01.002

Foucault, M. and Miskowiec, J. (1986) Of other spaces, *Diacritics*, 16(1): 22–7.

Goffman, E. (1961) *Asylums. Essays on the Social Situation of Mental Patients and Other Inmates*, Anchor Books.

Graverholt, B., Riise, T., Jamtvedt, G., Husebø, B. and Nortvedt, M.W. (2013) Acute hospital admissions from nursing homes: An example of unwarranted variation? *Scandinavian Journal of Public Health*, 41(4): 359–65.

Gubrium, J. (1975) *Living and Dying at Murray Manor*, St. Martin's.

Harrington, C., Choiniere, J., Goldman, M., Jacobsen, F.F., Lloyd, L., McGregor, M., et al (2012) Nursing home staffing standards and staffing levels in six countries, *Journal of Nursing Scholarship*, 44(1): 88–98.

Hauge, S. (2004) Jo mere vi er sammen, jo gladere vi blir? Ein feltmetodisk studie av sjukeheimen som heim [A fieldwork-based study of the nursing home as a home], doctoral dissertation, University of Bergen.

Hauge, S. and Heggen, K. (2008) The nursing home as a home: A field study of residents' daily life in the common living rooms, *Journal of Clinical Nursing*, 17: 460–67.

Høyland, K., Denizou, K., Baer, D., Evensmo, H.F. and Feragen, P.S. (2018) *Fra universelt utformede bygg til inkluderende områdeutvikling* [Health promoting urban design], SINTEF Academic Publishing.

Høyland, K., Kirkevold, Ø., Woods, R. and Haugan, G. (2015) *Er smått alltid godt i demensomsorgen? Om bo- og tjenestetilbud for personer med demens* [Is small always beautiful in dementia care? On housing and services for persons living with dementia], SINTEF Academic Publishing.

Jacobsen, F.F. (2015) Continuity and change in Norwegian nursing homes, in the context of Norwegian welfare state ambitions, *Ageing International*, 40: 219–22.

Jacobsen, F.F. (2014) De eldres integritet i en sykehjemskontekst [Integrity of older adults in the context of nursing home], in S. Stein Husebø, and M. Holm (eds) *Omsorg ved livets slutt – en verdig alderdom?* [End of life care – dignity in older age?], Fagbokforlaget, pp 363–72.

Jacobsen, F.F. (2015) De eldres integritet i en sykehjemskontekst [Integrity of older people in a nursing home context], in Holm, M.S. and Husebø, S. (eds) *En verdig alderdom: Omsorg ved livets slutt* [Dignity in older age: End of life care], Fagbokforlaget, pp 267–76.

Jacobsen, F.F. (2021) Sykehjemspraksiser i kontekst: Søkelys på romlige og fysiske forutsetninger og føringer [Nursing home practices in context: Highlighting spatial and physical conditions and constraints], in L. Kjersti and R. Horne (eds) *Praxeologiske perspektiver*, Hexis Publishing, pp 293–311.

Jacobsen, F.F., Arntzen, C., Devik, S.A., Førland, O., Krane, M. S., Madsen, L., et al (2021) *Erfaringer med COVID-19 i norske sykehjem: Underlagsrapport for Koronakommisjonen* [Experiences of COVID-19 in Norwegian nursing homes: A report for the Norwegian Corona Commission], Report 1/2021, Centre for Care Research.

Jacobsen, F.F. and Sundsbø, A.O. (2020) *Et aldersvennlig Norge* [Age-friendly surroundings and communities in Norway], Norwegian University of Science and Technology, Gjøvik, Omsorgsbiblioteket.

Lund, S. (2003) Hjemmekos: Iscenesettelse av norsk familiesamvær, *Norsk Antropologisk Tidsskrift*, 14(1): 27–34.

Löfqvist, C., Granbom, M., Himmelsbach, I., Iwarsson, S., Oswald, F. and Haak, M. (2013) Voices on relocation and aging in place in very old age – A complex and ambivalent matter, *The Gerontologist*, 53(6): 919–27.

Meagher, G. and Szebehely, M. (eds) (2013) *Marketisation in Nordic Eldercare*, Stockholm University.

Ministry of Health and Social Affairs (1996–97) 'Handlingsplan for eldreomsorgen. Trygghet – respekt – kvalitet' [Action plan for older people's care. Safety – respect – quality], White Paper No. 50, Norway Ministry of Health and Social Affairs.

Ministry of Social Affairs (2001–02) 'Avslutning av handlingsplan for eldreomsorgen' [Completion of the action plan for older people's care], White Paper No. 31, Norway Ministry of Social Affairs.

Munkejord, M. C., Eggebø, H. and Schönfelder, W. (2018) Hjemme best? Eldres fortellinger om omsorg og trygghet i eget hjem [Is living at home always best? Older people's stories about care and security in own home], *Tidsskrift for Omsorgsforskning*, 4(1):16–26.

Norwegian Broadcasting Corporation (NRK) (2022) 'Scotching the myth that older people just want peace and quiet and a panoramic nature view', Available from: https://www.nrk.no/vestland/avlivar-myten-om-at-eldre-berre-vil-ha-stille-og-naturutsikt-1.15834677

OECD (2022) 'Long-term care resources and utilization: Beds in residential long-term care facilities', *OECD.Stat*, Available from: https://stats.oecd.org/Index.aspx?QueryId=30142

Rostgaard, T., Jacobsen, F.F., Kröger, T. and Peterson, E. (2022) Revisiting the Nordic long-term care model for older people – still equal?, *Socio-Economic Review*, 18(3):725–43, doi: 10.1093/ser/mwy026

Statistics Norway (2020) 'Fire av fem eldre som dør, mottar omsorgstjenester i kommunen' [Four out of five older people who die receive long-term care services], Available from: https://www.ssb.no/helse/artikler-og-publikasjoner/fire-av-fem-eldre-som-dor-mottar-omsorgstjenester-i-kommunen

Statistics Norway (2021) 'Users of nursing and care services, by age and nursing and care service categories 2015–2020', Available from: https://www.ssb.no/en/statbank/table/12003/tableViewLayout1/

Stig, K., Paulsson Lütz, I., Erichsen, E., Palotie-Heino, T., Knape, et al (2013) *Financing of Healthcare in the Nordic Countries*, Nordic Medico Statistical Committee, Available from: https://norden.diva-portal.org/smash/get/diva2:968753/FULLTEXT01.pdf

10

Conclusion: a labour of love is still labour

Pat Armstrong, Hugh Armstrong and Marta Szebehely

The line between paid and unpaid work in nursing homes has become increasingly blurred. While values play a role, funding, ownership, staffing, the division of labour, and physical structures are also critical to understanding this development. Our research in Norway, in Sweden and in Ontario, Canada's largest province, shows how the boundaries between paid and unpaid work are shaped by these factors in ways that indicate the flexibility in expectations and demands for each kind of work. In all three countries, workloads for paid staff have increased at the same time as their employment has become more precarious. All three have experienced consequences from neoliberal approaches to care services and labour organisation. Nevertheless, the continuing Scandinavian commitment to a form of universalism, reflected in more funding for long-term care, less for-profit ownership, and higher staffing levels, as well as in more autonomy for staff and a less rigid division of labour, means there is much less unpaid work left to be done than in the Ontario case.

The blurred boundaries between paid and unpaid work are evident in the similarities between the two kinds of labour. Most obviously, the paid and unpaid work is done in the same workplace, and the boundaries are particularly blurred when the unpaid work is done by the people who are otherwise paid to do it. Working short when not everyone scheduled to work shows up has become common in all three countries, meaning that more work is done for the same pay and some paid work may remain undone. Especially in Ontario, where neoliberalism has the strongest hold of the three countries, staff go in early, work though breaks and lunch, and stay late, mostly without pay for their additional time on the job. Also mainly in Ontario, family, friends and volunteers undertake a significant amount of work within the nursing home to make up for the gaps in care.

For both kinds of workers, the unpaid labour spills out beyond the nursing home. In all three countries, paid staff take their work to their own homes, worrying about what care they left undone. But, again, this is most common in Ontario, where paid staff may also do unpaid laundry or shopping work for residents unpaid. Family, friends and volunteers may do some tasks outside the nursing home workplace, tasks such as arranging appointments, worrying, handling finances or taking residents on trips.

Both paid and unpaid work are shaped by the physical environment and the location of the home. Nursing homes located in settings and with structures that allow the outside community in and the inside community out support residents in providing self-care and enable families, friends, volunteers and even casual visitors to participate in activities and foster a sense of belonging. In offering multiple opportunities for social connections, this kind of integration can also help reduce the unpaid work required by staff. Private bedrooms and communal dining rooms can encourage families to visit, while good transportation can reduce the unpaid time staff and others spend getting to the home. In rural areas, distance can make it hard for families to provide unpaid care and small communities can mean that staff spend time outside the home addressing work issues raised by families and acquaintances.

In Ontario, those paid and not paid increasingly do the same tasks. Families and friends brush teeth and hair, assist with eating and walking, change beds and wash bums and even bathe residents, to name only some of the common tasks. By contrast, families in Scandinavia told us they resisted such unpaid labour, maintaining this was the job of paid workers.

Residents in all three countries do tasks for themselves, which provides them with a sense of dignity and control. However, the increasingly heavy workloads for staff often mean there is less time to support residents in providing their own self-care or in offering assistance to others. A growing focus on medical care by staff in these countries means that family, friends and volunteers are often left to do the essential social support and connecting work. By sharing tasks, especially in Ontario, where a much broader range of tasks is done by family, friends and volunteers, unpaid and paid workers are also sharing skills. This can mean that aspects of both kinds of work are perceived as requiring little formal knowledge. It can also cause tensions between paid and unpaid workers as paid staff struggle to have their skills recognised and protected, and unpaid workers try to ensure care is provided, often by doing tasks they did for residents when they lived in their private homes.

Of course, there are still significant differences between the two groups of workers. Paid workers are required to be in nursing homes at specific hours and for specific lengths of time to do specific tasks, risking formal discipline or even job loss if they fail to do the work. In all three countries, the increasing numbers of workers employed on a part-time or casual basis may feel particularly at risk, and that risk may push them to put in unpaid work time.

The same does not apply to unpaid workers, although many put in long and regular hours. In Ontario, staffing levels are much lower than in Scandinavia and there is considerably less expectation that care will be provided by paid staff. Indeed, many Ontario families and friends tell us they feel forced to be in the nursing home every day to do specific tasks at times dictated by the schedules of the nursing homes, otherwise the health of their relative would be at risk. These unpaid workers also risk being banned from the home for doing some tasks or for advocating in ways the management or staff find problematic.

Volunteers may have regular scheduled hours, but the consequences are significantly less severe than for paid workers if they don't show up. Irregularity in unpaid work sometimes makes it difficult for staff to plan their tasks, creating tensions between the two groups. At the same time, in all three countries the growing number of part-time and casual staff, along with increasing turnover rates, means that more paid staff have irregular hours too, and there is more unpaid work to be done by families in ensuring these casual and part-time employees know about the individual needs and preferences of residents.

There are also differences in the structures of power and control. In all three countries, most workers in the nursing homes are unionised. Collective agreements provide staff with some important rights. However, these rights are limited by funding and by neoliberal employment strategies that have increased reliance on part-time and casual workers. In Ontario, where unions have had only limited success in resisting for-profit ownership, many services are contracted out to non-unionised companies. However, in all these countries, there is a growing reliance on agency workers who do not belong to unions. The hierarchical work organisation in Ontario, and to some extent in Scandinavia, also means those who provide the bulk of the daily care have the least power. This may be particularly the case for the growing numbers of workers who are immigrants and/or racialised.

Those who do unpaid work do not have the same formal rights as unionised workers. In Ontario, the required residents' councils are intended to provide residents with input into the home's life. But in some homes we have studied, the members of residents' councils are often not participants in decision-making so much as recipients of information.

Family councils vary considerably, first in terms of whether they exist at all and second, in terms of the extent to which they are able to actively shape what happens in the nursing home. Our research with family councils suggests that the pandemic has pushed them to become more active and more demanding in terms of having a say in how homes are run and in the determination of family as well as resident rights. In Sweden and Norway, designated contact persons help ensure that residents and families have some continuing say in care and in the nursing home's care strategies. However, there are rarely any other formal structures for input into the functioning of the care home.

Both those who are paid and those who are not frequently feel compelled to do unpaid work. Women especially feel responsible and are held responsible for care that would otherwise be left undone. Both kinds of work can be rewarding when they bring pleasure and comfort from supporting others in appropriate ways, but the extent to which the work is rewarding depends in large measure on the conditions of work.

The necessary conditions that stood out in our research include sufficient staff, along with continuity and autonomy for staff, and more emphasis on social care and self-care for residents. These conditions also include a more supportive admission process, clearer guidelines on who can do what, when and with whom, along with an opportunity for effective input into those guidelines. This must be accompanied by continual educational opportunities to keep up with changing needs. Accessible communications systems are also important, as are opportunities for teamwork. At the same time, accessible care homes bring the community in and allow residents out, while private rooms not only limit infections but provide opportunities for private connections. All of these measures need the support of more funding and of public provision, eliminating for-profit care.

By understanding what residents, families, friends and volunteers do, as well as some of what paid staff do, as unpaid work, we can expose the forces that shape this work and the conditions as well as the relations under which unpaid work is done. And we can develop strategies and actions to ensure that necessary medical and social care are actually and consistently undertaken. Naming it work does not eliminate care – or love for that matter. Rather, it calls attention to what is required to keep the care and the love. Residents, staff, families and volunteers deserve no less.

Index